SEDUCTION LINES
HEARD 'ROUND THE WORLD AND ANSWERS YOU CAN GIVE:

A WORLD BOOK OF LINES

By **Sol Gordon**, Ph.D.

PROMETHEUS BOOKS

Buffalo, New York

SEDUCTION LINES HEARD 'ROUND THE WORLD AND ANSWERS YOU CAN GIVE. Copyright © 1987 by Sol Gordon. Illustrations © 1987 by Rita Fecher. All rights reserved. Printed in the United States of America. No part of this book may be used or reproduced in any manner whatsoever without written permission, except in the case of brief quotations embodied in critical articles and reviews. Inquiries should be addressed to Prometheus Books, 700 East Amherst Street, Buffalo, New York 14215.

92 91 90 89 88 87   6 5 4 3 2 1

Library of Congress Cataloging-in-Publication Data

Gordon, Sol, 1923-
' Seduction lines heard 'round the world and answers you can give.

    1. Courtship—Miscellanea. 2. Sex—Miscellanea.
I. Title.
HQ801.G595 1987   306.7'34   87-20460
ISBN 0-87975-405-2

SEDUCTION LINES
HEARD 'ROUND THE WORLD AND ANSWERS YOU CAN GIVE:
A WORLD BOOK OF LINES

INTRODUCTION

What is the *ultimate* line heard 'round the world?

"If you really love me, you'll have sex with me."

Response:

"If you really loved me, you wouldn't put this kind of pressure on me."
or
"You would even if I didn't love you, so what's the point?"
or
"Hey, that's a line. . . . I read it in Gordon's book."
or even
"I don't *really* love you . . . so I don't have to have sex with you."

Another line:

"You have nothing to worry about. I'll pull out in time."

If someone tells you not to worry, worry. When is the last time someone told you not to worry and you stopped? (It is especially true in this case, since pulling out even before the male ejaculates is *not* a safe or reliable birth control method. Very few people are aware of the fact that males "come" prior to the full ejaculation. This small amount of pre-orgasmic semen can contain millions of sperm. Any one of them can impregnate a woman. Withdrawal is better than nothing, but not a whole lot.)

By contrast, the "best" line in the 1930s was uttered by Jean Harlow in the movie *Hell's Angels:*

"Would you be shocked if I put on something more comfortable?"

One of the great responses of all times was made to George Bernard Shaw, the not very attractive English writer, who said to the gorgeous dancer Isadora Duncan:

"Let's you and I have an affair. With your body and my mind we'll have the world's most desirable baby."

Her reply:

"What if the child has my mind and your body?"

The best of current responses comes from a colleague, Dr. Sylvia Hacker. After having given a lecture on sex to a group of physicians, one approched and said:

"No need for preliminaries. Let's you and I have an affair."

Her response:

"Only if it's catered."

Remember: It's not romantic just to let it happen. It's stupid.

Warning: This book is not for females only.
This book of lines is for your amusement.
It will help you appreciate that sex is never a test or a proof of love.
There are cultural and ethnic differences in lines. The hundreds of clever responses will give you an edge on the "scene."
But, (especially) women, if you are alone and may be in danger of being raped, don't use a sarcastic or humiliating response that would enrage a potential rapist. Use your smarts to get out of a bad situation, possibly even screaming and fighting if you believe someone will come to your rescue or you can frighten the rapist away.
How did I collect the lines? Every semester during my fifteen

years at Syracuse University, I have taught a class on Human Sexuality to about five hundred students from all fifty states and many countries of the world. My students helped me collect thousands of lines.

    Dear reader,
How about dropping me a _____ ?

HOW CAN YOU TELL IF YOU'RE REALLY IN LOVE?

Many people confuse sex with love. Yet there are people who have enjoyable sex and who don't even like each other, and there are couples who love each other and whose sex lives are far from adequate but may be in a stage of very gradual development toward mutual satisfaction. About the dumbest thing anyone can do is to marry for sex or, as it is often called, chemistry. Even well-intentioned people say things to young people like, "If you have sex before marriage you'll have nothing to look forward to in marriage. There'll be no surprise in marriage." I say, if that's the only surprise in marriage, don't marry. It's not worth it.

Some say love is blind. I say it's blind for only twenty-four hours. Then you have to open up your eyes and see whom you are in love with. Love at first sight? Maybe, but better take another look.

The plain fact is that if you feel yourself to be in love, you are. However, there are two kinds of love: mature and immature. It's not difficult to tell the difference. Mature love is energizing. Immature love is exhausting. If you have an immature relationship, you have a tendency to be tired, you procrastinate a lot, you don't do your school work or your job well. You avoid your domestic responsibilities. (Me? Wash the dishes? I can't do that, I'm in love!) You have what we call a "hostile dependent relationship." You can't stand to be without the person you're supposed to be in love with ("I miss him," "I miss her," endlessly), but when you are together you fight and argue most of the time. Mood swings, accusations of jealousy, even violence characterizes the relationship. (Some people even confuse love and hate. If someone beats you up or forces sex upon you—that has nothing to do with mature love. You may think it's "love," but it's really stupidity or neurosis or dependency or fear.) In an immature relationship, one person usually says over and over again, "Do you love me? Do you really love me?" I advise the other person to say "no." You'll have your first real conversation that way.

Immature relationships are characterized by promises. "Don't worry, honey, when we get married I'll stop fooling around with other people." You might as well know now that a bad situation is *always* made worse by marriage. Immature relationships reveal insensitivity and selfishness by one or both persons, or that one person is trying to meet the needs of the other and both are not satisfied. Love feels like a burden.

Sally says she has a headache, but Don is angry and replies, "You have a headache on my day off. You have a lot of nerve." In a mature relationship, Sally's headache is responded to with, "I'm sorry you have a headache, honey. I'll get you an aspirin. There is always tomorrow."

Mature relationships are full of energy. You have time to do almost everything you want to. You don't shirk responsibilities. When you are together you enjoy each other. You might argue sometimes but not too much. You want to please each other. If you have a mature relationship, you are nice to other important people in your life—parents, younger siblings, and especially friends.

People who have immature relationships have a tendency to be mean to significant others in their life, especially friends. (Remember, lovers come and go—real friends are forever.) A good rule: Never give up a close, meaningful friendship for the sake of someone who might turn out to be only a temporary lover.

How can you tell if it's infatuation or mature love? The first month you can't. (In the summer it takes two months.) Infatuation and mature love appear and feel exactly the same. Once the relationship settles in, all or some of the above signs will appear, and you will be able to tell if you are *really* in love. Now some of you know why you are tired most of the time.

Some good general rules: Sex is never a test or proof of love. You can't buy love with sex. Many females have sex because of the possibility of love, but many more males have sex because of the possibility of sex. A large number of males find it easier to make out than to make conversation. I'm not anti-male, and I know that anything I've written about males is also true of some females. It's just that most males (not all, by any means) are programmed by society (not born) to exploit females.

So until such time as men and women stop playing games with each other, women had better be "good" at the games!

Of course we know that some relationships start out immature and with a lot of caring and effort become mature (and some start out mature and drift into anger and hostility). The key here is that mature relationships are an evolving—not always easy or magical—process.

I like what John Nelson says about love:

> Love is "a many-splendored thing." It is the desire for intimacy and the willingness to be vulnerable. It is rejoicing in the presence of the other, a commitment to the wider causes of the other. It is friendship. And it rests upon a solid sense of the self's own worth and, ultimately, upon a deep sense of cosmic acceptance, of being at home in the universe.
>
> from *Between the Gardens*
> by James Nelson
> New York: Pilgrim Press, 1983

Even if you decide that you really are in love, you don't have to have sex to prove it. The best test of a relationship is being able to hold off having sex until you both are ready and sure. There are lots of good ways of expressing affection—like making out, kissing, hugging, holding hands. If he or she says (upon your refusal to have sex):

"But that means you don't love me."

Your best response is:

"You are forcing me to have some second thoughts about it."

The bottom line is intimacy—getting to know and trust each other.

In fact, if I were to think of the ten most important aspects of a relationship, in order of importance, I would include:

1. Intimacy,

2. A sense of humor (please don't have any children if you don't have a sense of humor),
3. The ability to communicate your feelings to each other without hostility,
4. ⎫
5. ⎪
6. ⎬ (your own ideas)
7. ⎪
8. ⎭
9. Sexual fulfillment,
10. Sharing household tasks together.

One Final Caution:
- People flirt in order to get to know each other.
- People use lines in order to use (or exploit) each other.

AIDS ALERT

The line that was emerging as one of the most popular in the late 1980s:

"I just want to make you feel good"

is now quickly going out of style because of the fear of AIDS.

AIDS (Acquired Immune Deficiency Syndrome) is a fatal, contagious disease. It is, as of 1988, an incurable disease that cripples the immune system, leaving the victims susceptible to infections and cancers.

It is caused by a virus (not a sin) and is spread by sexual intercourse or exchange of blood (as in shared hypodermic needles). In the United States, most of the cases have been among homosexual and bisexual men. In Africa, most of the afflicted are heterosexuals. In any case, AIDS is spreading rapidly and increasingly among heterosexuals.

It may take five to nine years before symptoms appear. The main symptoms of AIDS include a persistent cough, high fever, and difficulty in breathing. Purplish blotches and bumps on the skin may indicate the development of cancer. Unfortunately, AIDS can be transmitted by someone who is infected but doesn't show symptoms. Anonymous blood tests for AIDS are available at clinics throughout the country.

For sexually active people the rule is now: "No sex without condoms." That includes anal, oral, and vaginal sex. AIDS is not transmitted by casual contact but mainly by sexual intercourse. So, "safer sex" means no sex without birth control for women and condoms for men. (Although we are concentrating here on AIDS, this guideline is good for prevention of all other venereal diseases and unwanted pregnancy.) So unless you are married to someone you are sure about, and you want babies—no sex without protection.

But, but, but, but, what if he says:

"If you really love me you'll have sex with me"?

Your response, if you love him and want to have sex with him, is:

"I really love you, but do you have a condom?"

He'll likely say,

"But, honey, I get no feeling from a condom."

Your immediate response:

"All the other men I know get plenty of feelings with condoms."

If he asks,

"What's the matter with you?"

Respond:

"Look, it's not easy, but we are into a real epidemic. We *have to* protect ourselves."

You could also start out by saying,

"The condom is my favorite protection. What's yours?" [At the same time, to protect against pregnancy, you use the pill or contraceptive foam.]

He might make a fuss and say:

"But I get so little pleasure when I wear a condom."

Your response is:

"In that case, you won't get any pleasure at all!"

He might ask:

"Does that mean you're not going to have sex with me?"

Your response has to be:

"You got it, buddy."

Men are not the only ones buying condoms these days. Responsible women are also buying condoms and using them as part of their sex play. The woman should put it on the man at the first signs of an erection—and be sure he holds onto it when he pulls out. (Do not use the same condom more than once.)

Warning: There is no such thing as safe sex. Only safer sex. Condoms are a big protection, but not a guarantee. Abstinence (no sex) is the only safe "sex." But abstinence does not mean you and the person you love have to sit at opposite ends of the room with your hands folded politely in your laps. You can still embrace and massage each other—hugs and kisses and mutual masturbation can be satisfying expressions of love.

For more information:
- *Center for Disease Control National Hotline:* Call toll free, 1-800-342-7514.
- *New York State Department of Health AIDS Hotline:* 1-800-541-2437.
- *National AIDS Hotline:* 1-800-634-7477.
- *Gay Men's Health Crisis Hotline:* 1-212-807-6655. (It's a toll call, but they're open 24 hours a day.)
- For the best information on safer sex ideas and techniques read The Institute for the Advanced Study of Human Sexuality's *The Complete Guide to Safe Sex,* published by Specific Press.
- For an especially up-to-date pamphlet on sexually transmitted disease, send one dollar to: American Foundation for the Prevention of Venereal Diseases, 799 Broadway, Suite 638, New York, N.Y. 10003.

My thirty-second Birth Control message: Listen, women, if you are not on the pill, be sure to use contraceptive foam. And if the guy can't afford fifty cents for a condom, he is too cheap to be allowed in!

And finally, the best line, which may not be a line at all:

"I like you. Can we talk?"

MOST POPULAR LINES IN THE 1980s

Haven't we met somewhere before?

You want it as much as I do.

If I told you you had a nice body, would you hold it against me?

Want to get high?

Want to go for a pizza and then have sex?
 No, get lost.
What's the matter, you don't like pizza?

Sit on my lap and we'll talk about the first thing that comes up.

Hey, get your Jordache jeans over here.

Would you like to dance?
 No.
Then I guess a blow job's out of the question.

BEST RESPONSES IN THE 1980s

What if he says,

> "Once you start, you can't stop"?

Just say,

> "I think I hear my boyfriend coming."

He'll stop in a second. And if he says,

> "I'll go crazy if we don't."

Reply:

> "Go." (No male has ever died from an unrelieved erection. The best cure for "blue balls" is masturbation.)

He: "You can't just leave me hanging like this after leading me on this far."
She: "Want to bet?"

He: "Would you like to party [meaning sex, drugs, and alcohol]?"
She: "No party, smarty."

Get a load of this one . . .

He: "Oh, oh, (desperate) I'll just stay in for a minute!"

She: (relaxed) "What do you think I am, a microwave oven?" (Humor reduces the erection instantly!)

He: "Oh, honey, I just want it to be spontaneous."
She: "Who are you kidding? You've been planning this for months."

LINES HEARD IN THE UNITED STATES AND SOME CLEVER RESPONSES

SMART RESPONSE LINES

Haven't we met before?
Yes, the V.D. clinic, wasn't it?

Hey, foxy mama, what's that gleam in your eye?
Disgust!

Your hair color is fabulous.
Thank you. It's on aisle three at the corner drug store.

Want to play strip poker?
Sorry, you haven't got the ante!

Hey, good lookin', can I buy you a drink?
Do you know your fly is open?

You look like a dream.
Go back to sleep.

I can tell that you want me.
Yes, I want you to leave.

I don't have any luck with women.
Well, perhaps you should try having a conversation with one.

Oh, you smell so good.
At least someone around here does.

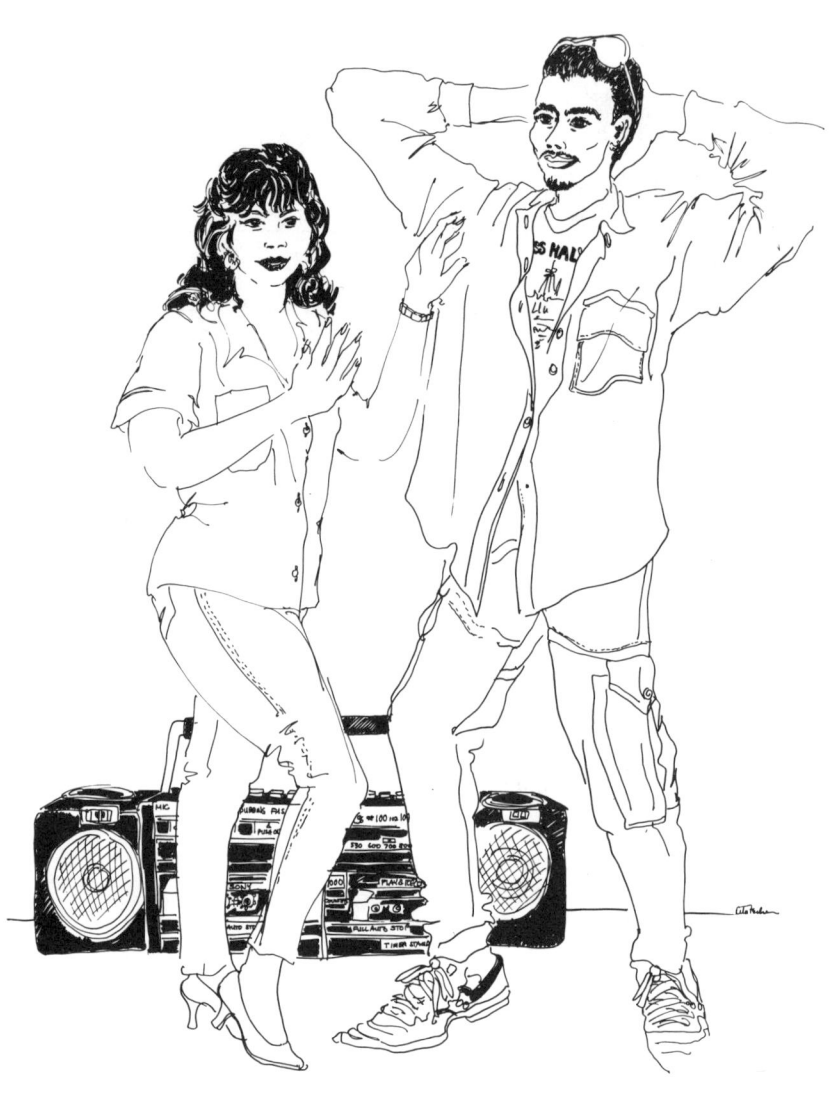

He: I'm well known; you must have seen me in the movies.
She: Where do you usually sit?

Hey, baby, what's your sign?
> *Do not enter.*
>> or
> *Stop.*

What course are you taking?
> *Everything except intercourse.*

Let's go for a walk and look at the foliage.
> *Make like a tree and leave.*

We can talk body language.
> *You can talk to somebody else.*

I want to give myself to you.
> *Sorry, I don't accept cheap gifts.*

From me, you can have anything you want.
> *Privacy.*

Hey, I'm a geology major; do you want to come over and see my rocks?
> *No, thanks, I'd rather stay home and get stoned!*

If you were a streetcar named Desire, I'd never get off.
> *I'm too fast for you to ride.*

May I see you pretty soon?
> *Don't you think I'm pretty now?*

I'd go through anything for you.
> *Let's start with your bank account.*

May I have the last dance?
> *You've just had it.*

May I hold your hand?
> *No thanks, it isn't heavy.*

Say you love me, say you love me.
> *"You love me."*

I'm well known; you must have seen me in the movies.
Where do you usually sit?

I would go to the end of the world for you.
Yes, but would you stay there?

I like the perfume you are wearing. What is it?
Untouchable.

If you give me a back rub, I'll give you one.
Sorry, you rub me the wrong way.

But if you don't go to bed with me, it'll force me to homosexuality.
Would you like to meet my brother then?

I just want to show you how much I love you.
Save the show and stick to the tell.

You know I'd never do anything to hurt you.
That's funny, what do you think this does?

Would you like to go outside for some air?
What are we breathing in here?

If you really love me, you will show me.
I'll show you, right to the door!

I've never felt like this before. I think I am in love.
I've never felt like this before either. I am getting depressed.

You are a very talented person. You dance like a butterfly.
You are not bad either. You managed to keep my shoes intact.

You're special; you're different; you're everything I want in a woman.
Your vocabulary is improving. Last time it was: You're something else, something I'll never find in any other woman.

When I look into your dark eyes, when I look at your dark silky hair, I lose myself in your beauty.
Maybe you should buy a flashlight.

My God, how angelic your face looks. It is true what they say, that when angels are present, devils disappear.
I see that you're still here.

My poetic talent erupted when I first set eyes on you.
I am sorry, but I was thinking of meeting someone more stable.

I've been watching you all night. You are the most beautiful girl in the room.
Thanks, keep watching.

I'll respect you in the morning.
Good then, I'll see you tomorrow.

You have such a wonderful glow. Where are you from?
Three Mile Island.

Mmmm, what's that cologne?
Schlitz.
    or
Pest repellent, and it's not working.

I could show you things you've never seen.
What you have probably wouldn't interest me.

Have you ever made love to a perfect stranger?
Nobody's perfect.

Want to have oral sex?
Yeah, let's just talk about it.

I bet I can find your G spot.
I don't think so, my apartment is a mess.

Your lips are very desirable.
Watch closely and read them, "Get lost!"

My balls ache, and only you can relieve the pain.
Okay, if you think that slapping you in the face will help.

Your place or mine?
> *Both. You go to your place, and I'll go to mine.*

All talk, no action.
> *I'll fix that. How about no talk and no action—goodbye.*

Come with me. I want to be your best friend.
> *I'm my own best friend.*

I would love to know what comes between you and your Calvins.
> *Nothing gets between me and my Calvins.*

Sex isn't such a big deal. What are you waiting for?
> *I'm waiting for someone it's a big deal with.*

You can't leave me this way.
> *Watch me!*

Your body is like a temple.
> *Sorry, there are no services today.*

WOE IS ME LINES

I've had such a hard day.
I understand, honey. I can see you're not up to making love.

You wouldn't want to hurt my feelings, would you?
Better that than my reputation.

I'm so depressed. I need someone to comfort me.
There's a very good psychologist at the other end of the bar.

I have this problem about meeting girls. I don't know what to say—could you help me?
Sure. You just say "Goodbye!"

You're really letting me down!
I guess you got yourself up for nothing.

No one ever can understand me. You look like you could understand and come to know me as I truly am.
Well, if you would sober up, your grammer would improve, and then more people could begin to understand you.

I have disappointment after disappointment these days, so don't let me down by saying that you won't come home with me.
Okay, I won't say it, but I won't come home with you either.

My girl threw me out. I have nowhere to go.
That's true.

I can't believe I'm so drunk. Please help me sober up.
> *Sure, I'll make you a thermos of coffee, and you can drink it on your way home—in the taxi.*

It is so tough being an only child. I've really led such a lonely life. Can you help remedy this terrible situation?
> *Well, I am twenty-three years old, but if your parents want to adopt me, I'll see what I can do.*

Here I am in a bar alone on my birthday, my girlfriend left me, my friends are all gone...
> *Better luck next year!*

What's the matter? I'm not good enough for you?
> *Bingo!*

Everyone expects so much from me. My wife, my kids, my boss and friends. Can't we just have a nice and relaxing relationship? You know. A free and easy time, with no ties.
> *Oh absolutely. You send me Christmas cards once a year, and I'll send postcards to you and your loved ones on my next cruise.*

But every other girl I've ever gone out with has said yes. . . .
> *Just because you're going out with me doesn't mean you're coming in!*

But, honey, it'll only take a little while!
> *That's the problem, it always only takes a little while!*

DIRECT LINES

In case you haven't noticed, I'm making it perfectly obvious that I want to go to bed with you.

I think you are the most beautiful girl in the place, and I would like to get to know you better.

God, what a meat market this place is. I'm really glad I'm not like all those other guys.

Excuse me. Do you see that guy over there? He's gay and has been following me around all night. [Putting his arm around her.] Could you please play along until he gets the message? Please?

So many girls say "no" when they mean "yes."
  When I mean "yes," you'll know.

You bring out the animal in me.
  I never wanted the animal—just the person.

I'd like to make it with you.
  Thanks, but I'm sure you'll make it fine on your own.

I really want to be your first.
  Sorry, you're about two years too late.

Would you like to make love?
  Out of what?

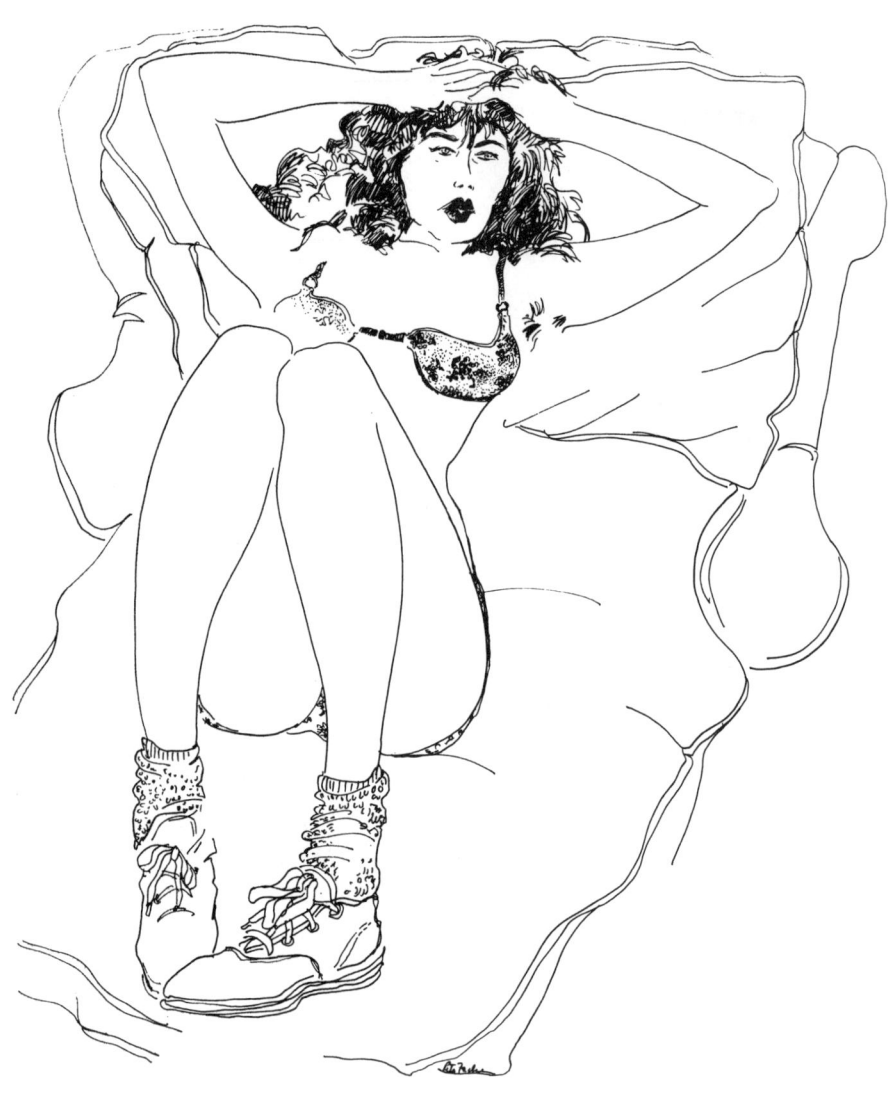

In case you haven't noticed, I'm making it perfectly obvious that I want to go to bed with you.

Don't worry; I'll pull out.
> *I'm not worried; you won't pull in.*

Let's make love together.
> *I've heard it's more fun by yourself.*

I've been told by many girls that I'm great in bed. Would you care to join me tonight?
> *No thanks. Most girls lie.*

What's your sign?
> *Radioactive.*

Make like a door knob and give me a turn.
> *Make like a baby and head out.*

What are you doing after work?
> *Teaching a karate lesson.*

I have a waterbed. Want go to for a swim?
> *Why? You're already all wet.*

Let's play carnival; sit on my face, and I'll guess your weight.
> *Carnival's great! Stand against the wall, and I'll throw baseballs at your head.*

Haven't I slept with you before?
> *Not unless you moonlight as a stuffed bear.*

Why are you trying so hard to ignore me?
> *Believe me, I don't have to try!*

It's been a great evening, let's end it "right."
> *Yes, right now.*

How about a b-job.
> *Do you have a condom?*

Hey gorgeous, can I buy you a drink?
> *You can buy me as many drinks as you want, just as long as you don't talk to me or make it look as if you know me.*

What ya drinking?
> *Cyanide. Want some?*

Well, baby, this is going to be your lucky day.
> *You mean you're going to leave me alone?*

Can't we go someplace and do it just a little?
> *Sure, if you can promise I'll only get pregnant a little.*

Is this seat empty?
> *Yes, and this one will be too if you sit down.*

I like the way you kiss.
> *Good, now please stop drooling all over me.*

I love fast women.
> *I love patient men.*

Come on, who'll know?
> *I'll know.*

What's it like being the most beautiful girl in the bar?
> *What's it like being the biggest liar in the world?*

I've got no place to stay tonight, mind if I stay with you?
> *Sure. Here's a pillow, here's a blanket, and there's the floor.*

RUDE AND CRUDE LINES

Wanna dance?
   No.
Then is a blow job out of the question?

Would you like to play with my heat-seeking moisture missile?

Is that a roll of quarters in your pocket, or are you just happy to see me?

Hey, bitch, how about a little chocha?

Give me a rim job, lady.

Hey, you want to get poked?

Give me a little Ock tonight, baby.

I'm an excellent gardener, so let me take care of that bush.

Hey, boot, ya wanna get polished?

How would you like to play find the monkey?
   What monkey?
The hairy monkey in my pants.

My pet snake is looking for a dark hole to crawl into.

I feel like a volcano about to burst. Baby, you can catch my lava when it flows.

Do you want to see my circumcision scar?

Can I have a blow job?
> *Sorry, I don't do miniatures.*

Want to see my one-eyed trouser mouse?
> *Yes, I'd like to feed it rat poison.*

I want to stick my dick where the sun doesn't shine.
> *So stick it in a closet.*

Oh, excuse my hard-on.
> *Put that little thing away.*

Why don't you come over to my place and show me the real curves?
> *I already have one ass in my pants, and I don't need another.*

Can I tickle your ass with a feather?
> *What? Did you say, "Pretty foul weather"?*

How about swallowing some sperm?
> *No thanks, I'm on a salt-free diet.*

How about a quickie?
> *O.K. Hurry up and leave.*

Hey, why don't you come back to my place? I heard you were easy.
> *I heard you can't get hard!*

What would you say to a little fuck?
> *Hi, little fuck.*

MUSICAL LINES

Bass players use their base instincts.
You've just sunk lower than your instrument.

Do you want to come to my room and see my organ?
No thanks. You can play it by yourself.

Haven't you heard that drummers have great rhythm?
Beat it.

I'll let you fiddle with my baton.
No way. You can't even conduct yourself.

Do you like Bach?
Sure, just as long as you don't Handel me.

I'll let you play my G-string.
Forget it, it's flat anyway.

We can make beautiful music together.
O.K., but only if you play your own instrument.

Let's go to my room. I'll teach you how to play the French horn.
Sorry pal, you'll have to blow your own horn.

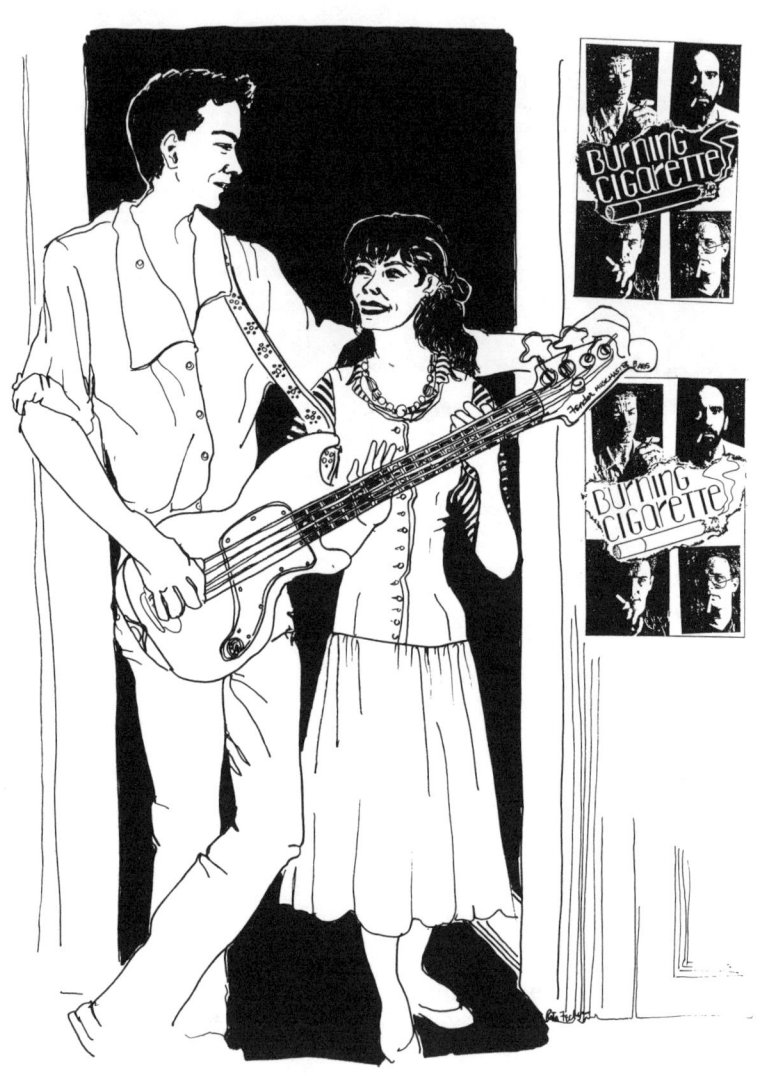

He: We can make beautiful music together.
She: O.K., but only if you play your own instrument.

LINES FROM ROCK 'n ROLL SONGS

(Clash): Should I stay, or should I go?
You should definitely go.

(REO Speedwagon): I saw you at midnight in a dream that I had.
Wake up and face reality.

(Olivia Newton-John): Let's get physical.
No thanks, I'm not into S and M.

(Police): I can't stand losin' you.
You never had me.

(Doors): Come on, baby, light my fire.
I heard you're out of fluid.

(La Belle): Voulez voux coucher avec moi ce soir?
I don't speak French.

(Air Supply): I'm lost without you.
I'll get you a compass.

(Lynard Skynard): What's your name, little girl?
I'm not a little girl; I'm a woman.

(Joan Jett): Do you wanna touch?
No thanks, I've got a weak stomach.

(Rick Springfield): I can make love a work of art.
   Yeah, I hear abstract art is really in.

(John Cougar Mellankamp): Come on make it hurt so good.
   No, I'm afraid I'll get hair in my braces.

(Rolling Stones): Let's spend the night together.
   I've got better plans.

(Earth, Wind and Fire): Would you mind if I make love to you till I'm satisfied?
   No thanks, I don't have that much time.

(Olivia Newton-John): I'm the one you want.
   That's funny, you don't look like _____ .

(Pat Benatar): I need a lover. . . .
   Why don't you establish a relationship first?

(Rod Stewart): Tonight I'm yours.
   No, I don't accept charity.

PREPPY LINES

My alligator is bigger than your alligator.

Want to wrestle alligators?

Stock Market trading is the most fun you can have with your clothes on!

Do you want to bag some ZZZs with me?

How about a little tongue sushi?

That's a nice Faire Isle you're wearing.

What do you think about the merger between DuPont and Sunoco?

You look like you own a Mercedes? Do you?

Can I take a bite out of your alligator?

I really like your alligator.
   Watch out; it bites.

RHYME LINES

What's cookin', good-lookin'?

Sex at a fast rate, keeps you in great shape.

You're so sweet, every time I look at you my heart skips a beat.
 Give me a treat and let it skip a beat.

Look, I know you want to stay tonight.
 I know that even though you failed to score, perhaps you'll learn that less is more.

Hey, Honey! I have meat that is a real treat.
 Well, you'd better take a back seat, because it is no feat, to have a treat that is so petite.

Let's go dancin' and prancin', romancin' and depantsin'.
 Find a sheep you can keep who won't breathe a peep if you take her to sleep, you miserable creep.

JOCK LINES

I noticed your goal post; your end zone isn't bad either.

Would you like to make love—and not on the courts?

My jersey may be 69, but I can play any position.

I see you're a relay runner. Do you handle all sticks well?

Hey, aren't you on the football team? I'd recognize that "bod" anywhere.

Oh, you're on the track team—want to go for a run up to my room?

I'd love to go for a run with you, but I have this awful muscle cramp in my thigh, and it really needs a massage. . . .

You play basketball? I bet I could dribble your balls real well.

I bet I can score on the first down.
   Not if I'm in my first period.

I bet you've been around the bases.
   Yes, but never in the same game with you.

How would you defend against a long pass, baby?
   With a tight prevent defense.

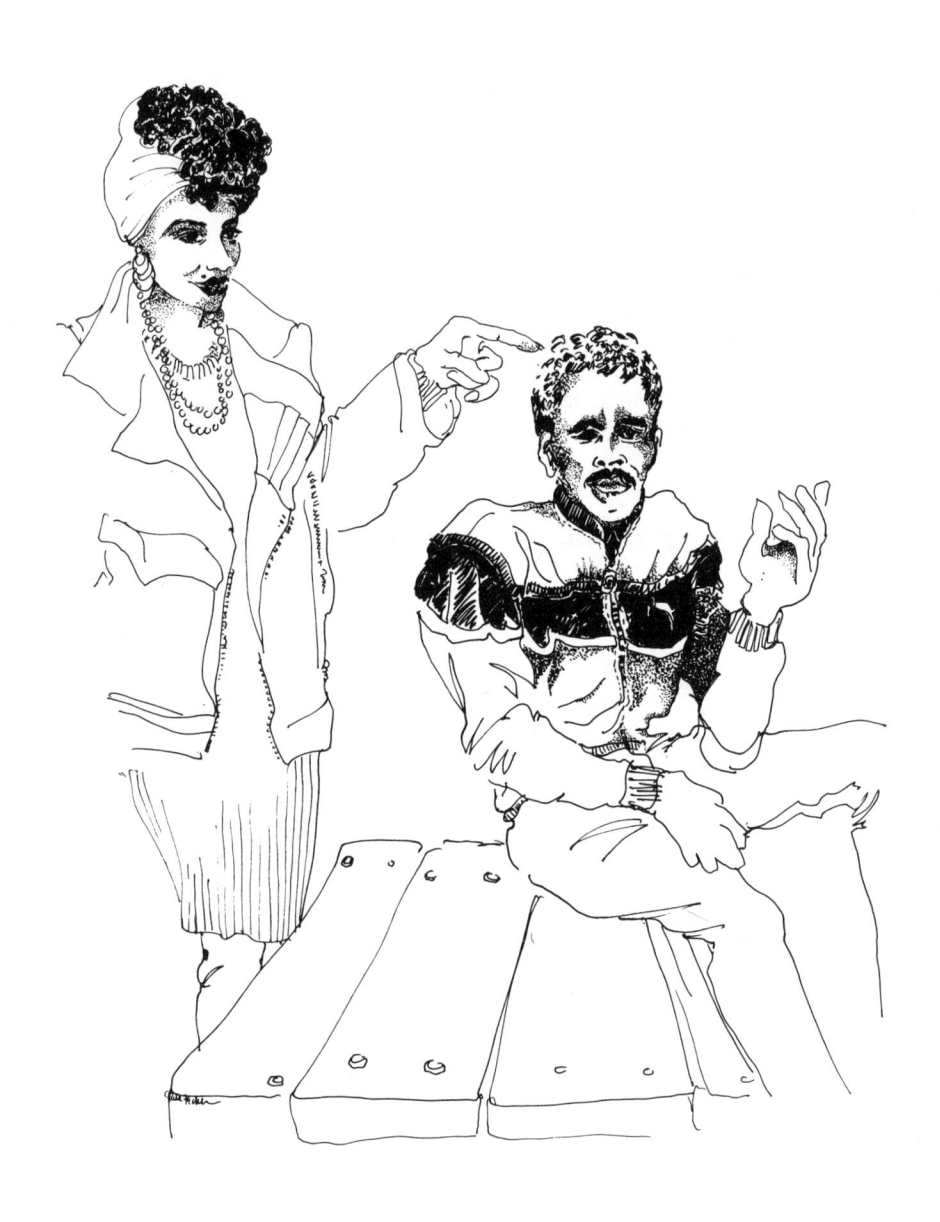

He: It takes a lot to develop all these muscles. How about you and me going to my place tonight, and I'll show you what it takes.
She: Well, I might, except that it looks like you've neglected the most important muscle of all.

Well, in that case, I'll just try another short pass.
> *Too bad for you it's fourth down and long yardage!*

How would you like to see me perform a back door, 360 degree slam dunk?
> *As long as you stay away from the rim when you shoot.*

Don't worry, I never get caught goaltending.
> *Well, I think I'll play defense just the same.*

Can I shoot my puck into your goal?
> *Only if your stick is protected.*

I've got some moves and positions to put you into.
> *But if you don't wear head-gear, you're disqualified.*

If you think these muscles are developed, you should see the ones I use under the covers.
> *Oh, I always wondered how you got such large, firm wrist muscles.*

It takes a lot to develop all these muscles. How about you and me going to my place tonight, and I'll show you what it takes.
> *Well, I might, except that it looks like you neglected the most important muscle of all [points to head].*

I play football; I've got great hands.
> *You just fumbled!*

Let's go to my place, and I'll show you some fancy moves.
> *The pass you just made is incomplete. Bye!*

I'll show you some backfield motion you'll never forget.
> *I'll penalize you for illegal use of hands.*

I'm fast and powerful in bed too!
> *Get the puck out of here!*

How about you and me getting into a little slam dunk action?
> *What would be a foul shot.*

When I bowl I always get a strike.
> *Spare me!*

In tennis, love is part of the score.
> *That line won't get you any points!*

SCOUT LINES

Let's tickle.

I'll show you mine if you show me yours.

You dig me. I dig you.

A bird in the hand is worth two in the bush.

Can I light your fire?
No, but you can go collect firewood.

Wanna have some fun tonight?
Sure, let's make some popcorn.

What are you doing tonight?
Come on over and we'll play monopoly.

Do you play games?
Would you like to play backgammon in my room?

UNCOMMON RESPONSES TO COMMON LINES

Haven't I seen you someplace before?
Yeah, that's why I don't go there anymore.

I remember you.
I forgot you.

Can I buy you a drink?
No, but you can buy one for my boyfriend; he's short on cash.

I promise I'll respect you in the morning.
Why don't you start by respecting me now?

If you don't, you'll be sorry—I'm a great catch.
The only problem is that I wouldn't know what I'd be catching.

I really like your style.
That's sweet. If you had some I'd probably like yours too.

Don't worry, I've got protection.
I hope it's from you.
   or
You're going to need protection if you get any closer.

Let's go back to my place and learn about each other.
Let's not and remain very vague.

YES AND NO LINES

Haven't I seen you somewhere before?
Why, yes.

I respect you. Why don't you have sex with me?
I respect my body too. That's why I won't have sex with you.

Want to see my apartment? I've got a great fireplace.
O.K., but you'd better keep your poker to yourself.

Do you like jocks like me?
No, I've never been an athletic supporter.

I may only have six inches, but some girls like it that thick.
Do you want to have sex, or do I owe you an apology?

Surely, surely you want to do it as badly as I do.
No, I don't, and stop calling me Shirley.

But every other girl I've ever gone out with has said yes.
Just because you're going out with me doesn't mean you're coming in.

ENGINEERED LINES

Hi, I'm a heat pump. May I engage myself in your wall?
Sorry, I'm non-supporting.

Your face is like a perimeter hydronic heat system—radiant.
And you remind me of a gas-fired sectional furnace—a lot of hot air!

I've erected some beauties in my day.
All low-rise, I suppose.

Have you ever seen a doric column?
Of course, I had a doll house once.

Would you mind if I slipped my tongue into your groove?
Sorry, I'm made of metal decking.

Could I fill your expansion joint with my neopreme stick?
Only if it's rubber coated.

Just set yourself on my concrete foundation.
If that's going to do the job, it's going to need quite a bit of reinforcing.

May I enter your honorific space?
That's last in the hierarchical sequence.

I like a girl without a false facade.
Oh really? I was wishing you had a brick veneer.

In case of emergency, may I break your fire box?
Sugar, with your equipment, you couldn't even scratch my glass.

Would you like to slide down my fire pole?
In case of fire, I'll take the stairs.

Honey, you *are* on fire. Let me hose you down.
Sorry, false alarm.

Do your mechanical systems need manual control?
Sorry, they're on automatic.

Hi, I'm a stud. Would you marry me?
Why don't you support a wall instead?

Would you like to inspect my stress points?
No need, I'm sure they'd fail.

LINES USED BY FEMALES

Would you like to seduce me?

Don't you think it would be a lot more comfortable if we went up to your room and stretched out a bit so we could talk and I could get to know you better?

I'm great at giving back massages, but only if you take off your shirt. How about it?

In case you haven't noticed, I'm making it perfectly obvious I want to go to bed with you.

Don't worry, I'm safe tonight. I took one of my mother's pills.

Sex makes you more of a ladies' man.

Sex makes your penis grow.

Sex builds up your muscles.

Sex makes your hair grow.

My parents are out of town, and I'm so afraid of staying here all by myself.

I'm much too tired to walk all the way back to my place—why don't we stop off at yours for a while first?

You're not trying to seduce me, are you?

Do you have the Bio notes on muscles?

Weren't you in my class last year?

Don't be afraid. You can touch any part of my body.

Do you want to come home with me tonight?

Do you want a massage?

You're the only one I could ever really love!

I'm getting my friend tomorrow.

Want to see my scar?

Are you ticklish?

Can I buy you a drink?

Are you interested in a one night stand?

Baby, you're not just another dick in the crowd.

Isn't sex great with strangers?

I just bought a vibrator; we can do all kinds of things with it.

Hi buddy. Wanna screw?
    No thanks, I've got a drawer full at home.

I've been around. I could show you a few things.
    If you've been around, you'd better keep going.

You should be flattered; I don't give my body up to anyone.
    I wouldn't want to ruin your record.

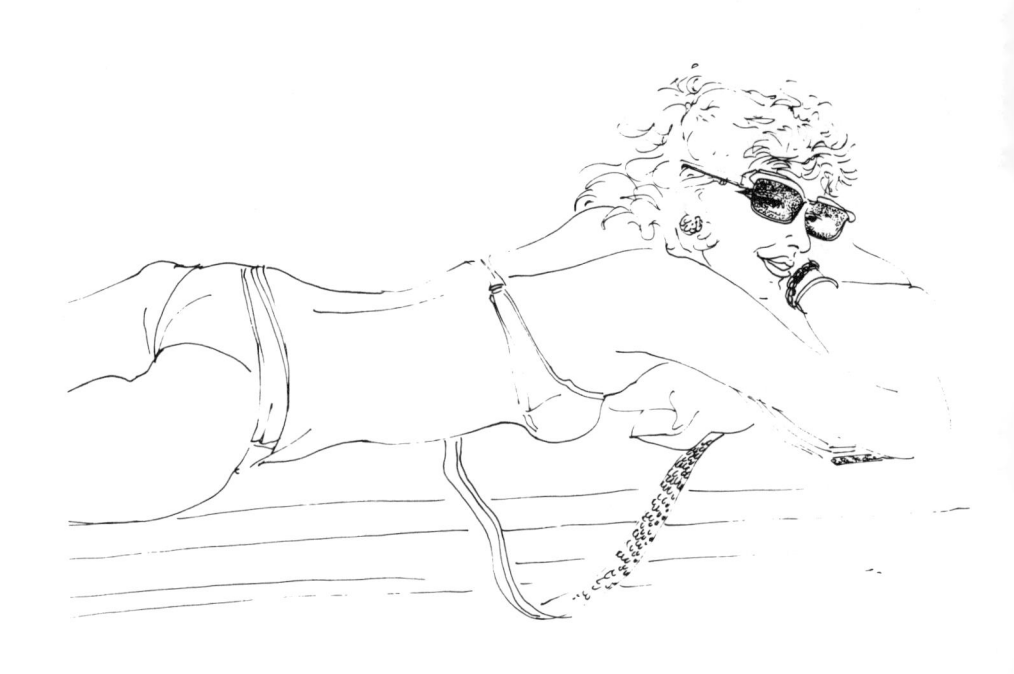

You're not trying to seduce me, are you?

I think sex is such an intimate thing. How about you?
Intimate enough not to do with you.

If you do it with me, I'll show you something you've never seen: multiple orgasms.
Oh, you can too; so do all my other women.

Baby, you could get lucky tonight if you play your cards right.
Yeah, maybe I'll win some money.

I love men who are frank.
Too bad, my name is Joe.

Will you join me?
Why, are you coming apart?

I was in a jam last night.
Tell me about it, but don't spread it too thick.

Are you trying to pick me up?
No, you're much too heavy.

How can my life be so confused and a mess? I'm only twenty years old. I guess I just need a man to help me through these times.
You are right, with that kind of thinking you show how messed up you really are. Who needs a loser?

Where have you been all my life?
Hiding from you!

NATURE LINES

Let's just be natural.

Good exercise, nature's many arousals, a climb to the climax, and beautiful scenery—what more could a guy ask for?

If you like those stalagmites and stalagtites, why don't you come over here and check out my formations?

Baby, c'mon over here and rest on my rocks.
  Thanks anyway, this rock's soft enough for me.

Let's go into the woods and make a beautiful scene.
  But why make more beautiful scenes when we haven't seen all the ones out here?

If you zip your sleeping bag to mine, you can be twice as warm.
  But then where would you sleep?

I want to do something no one has ever done down here—make love.
  Great, there's no problem finding you a Horny Bat.

Making love is like rowing a canoe, you just move over the rocks with a light hand on the paddle and move with the flow.
  Oh, you mean I have to pant and puff and work and moan and pretend it's feeling good for you to have a good time?

VEGETARIAN LINES

May I pick your cherry?
It isn't ripe yet.

May I squeeze your peaches?
No, you might bruise them.

Would you like your tomato stuffed?
Yes, but I don't think you have enough stuffing, so go stuff it somewhere else!

Hi, would you like to juice my carrot?
Yes, let's get my food processor!

EYE LINES

I noticed you staring at me from across the bar.
> *I didn't realize I was staring at you. Let me put my glasses on and see what I am supposed to be staring at.*

Your eyes are sparkling.
> *They only sparkle when I'm bored.*

Where did you get such gorgeous eyes?
> *They were on sale, two for a dollar.*

Do you know that you have bedroom eyes?
> *I know that I have bedroom nays.*

Your eyes are enough to bring a strong man to his knees!
> *So why are you still standing?*

If I look at your eyes any longer, I'm going to go crazy!
> *How will you be able to tell?*

Those sexy eyes tell me what you're thinking.
> *If you think I think you're full of shit, you're absolutely right!*

CLOTHES LINES

If I could see you naked, I'd die happy.
If I could see you naked, I'd die laughing.

I like your shirt. I'd love to see how it looks off of you.
Really? You can do my laundry any time.

I would really like to see the inside of those jeans.
Go to the shopping center. They've got thousands of them you can look at.

Do you, by any chance, have a black lace bra?
No, but you're going to have a black eye if you don't watch out!

LET'S PLAY LINES

Hey, want to join me?
I did not know you were falling apart.

Let's play Pinocchio: You sit on my face, and I'll tell you lots of lies.
I don't believe in fairy tales.

Let's play battleship: I'll lie down, and you blow the hell out of me.
How about if I just blow you out of my life?

Let's play golf: I'm sure I could get a hole-in-one.
Try it and I'll break your putter!

Let's play electrician: You turn on the juice, and I'll plug in my hot wire.
I'm afraid you've already burned out your fuse.

Hey, beautiful, want to come home with me?
I can't—I'm on my menstrual cycle.
    or
That's okay . . . you can follow me on my Honda.

MACHO LINES

Essentially, I'm doing you a favor by talking to you.

Mine's eight inches.
Don't worry, some people find big noses attractive.

Some girls say I remind them of a Hollywood movie star.
I knew it. I told my friend you were E.T. the minute I saw you, but she didn't believe me.

Say, baby, how would you like to go out with a very handsome, intelligent guy?
Oh, you have a friend?

Hey, baby, want the best you ever had?
Where would I find it?

I just got back from Hollywood where I made a movie called *The Stud*. Come with me and you'll learn the true meaning of the word.
I knew you looked familiar; I could have sworn, however, that the name of the movie was The Jerk.

I know how to please a woman.
Then please leave me alone.

I'll make you a new woman.
What's wrong with me now?

Nobody can give you what I can.
If it's V.D., you can keep it.

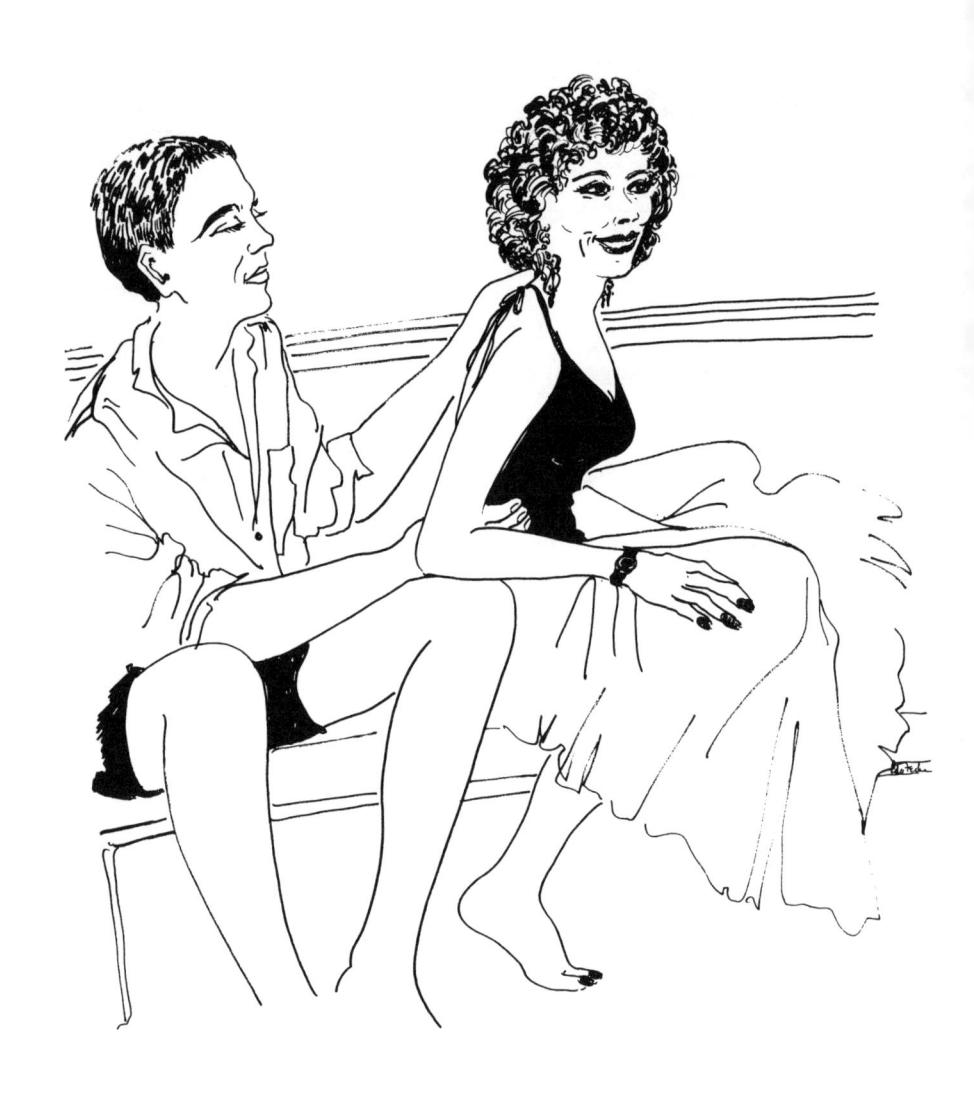

He: I know how to please a woman.
She: Then please leave me alone.

I consider my looks one of my greatest assets.
I'd hate to see your lesser ones.

No woman has ever rejected me.
Well, they had to make money somehow.

Hey, baby, I'm packing ten inches.
Yeah, those are very long feet.

When was the last time you saw a body like this?
Last night, while I was watching "The Flintstones" on T.V.

I'll make you feel like a million dollars.
That's how much you'll need to cover medical expenses if you touch me!

LINES OF LITERARY GENIUS

Was it something said? . . . Something done? . . .

We really museth, my darling, for you do realize that the inaudible and noiseless foot of time is upon us.
> *But I thought that you said that age cannot wither nor custom stale my infinite variety?*

But, my sweet, the ripest fruit first falls.
> *If you can't wait until harvest, you're not worth it.*

You don't have to think about it, sweetie. The woman who deliberates is lost.
> *Baby, the woman who doesn't deliberate has five kids and no alimony.*

Gather ye rosebuds while ye may/ Old Time is still a flyin'/ And this same flower that smiles today/ Tomorrow will be dyin'.
> *No problem, I'm kind of partial to silk roses myself, and they last forever.*

Come over here, prissy one. How many times have I told you that prudence in a woman should be an instinct not a virtue?
> *My best instincts right now, buddy, tell me to get out of here!*

Let's get comfortable!
> *It depends how* Great *your* Expectations *are, Charlie.*

Oh, my love, what's mine is yours and what's yours is mine.
> *Oh good! I'll take the Cadillac, the business, and the stocks! You can have the kitchenware that you gave me for Christmas!*

Believe me! My heart is true as steel.
> *If I were you, I'd put on some tennis shoes so when lightning strikes you'll be a better conductor!*

How much more elder art thou, than thou looks.
> *If age counts to you, buddy, you're either too young to know or too old to care.*

Yes, I am, ay, every inch a king.
> *You are using the centimeter side.*

DONCHA REALLY WANNA LINES

Where have you been all my life?
Dating real *people.*

It will be different with *me.*
Different doesn't mean better.

You don't know what you've been missing.
You won't know either.

You *know* you want it.
Too bad you don't know what it is I want.

Baby, I can be a real animal.
Sorry, I don't go for lower primates.

There's so much I want to give you.
V.D. isn't something I look forward to.

Try it this once—if you don't like it we'll never do it again.
If I try it now with you, I'm sure I'll never want to do it again.

There's so much I want to learn about you.
How about starting with this: When I say no, I mean no.

Could it be that I'm the one you've been waiting for?
Does hell freeze over?

Oh, come on! We've been through so much together. . . .
Yes, and you'd think by now you would understand me.

I know how to please women.
Maybe one day you'll learn to care about them.

ABSURD LINES

Let's go stoke the furnace, lady.
   Why bother when the coals are dead?

Do you want to hear about the rise and fall of the Roman Empire?
   It crumbled, didn't it?

Let's do some pushin' on the cushins.
   No, I'm afraid you'll find the latex in my Playtex.

Do you want to do this hard or easy?
   I wouldn't have thought you could get hard.

Let me show you how much I love you.
   First show me how much ice cream you can eat.

Did you ever make love on a golf course?
   Why, are you tee'd off?
      or
   No, golf shoes make permanent scars.

Want to jog around the shower?
   No, my raincoat is at the cleaners.

PRIVATE PARTY LINES

I've got a really nice pad.
I want a prince, not a frog.

I've got some great weed in my room.
Great! Why don't you go home, smoke about twenty joints, and fantasize about me.

Want to come to my apartment and see my record collection?
It might be fun, but I don't want to become part of your record.

Would you like to see the house?
John showed it to me already, thank you.

Would you like to go to my room, where it is more quiet, and smoke a joint?
No thank you. I like the noise down here.

I have better drinks up in my room. Would you like to have some?
No thanks. I'm already drunk.

Why don't we have our own little party up in my room?
The party is great down here.

I'm holding a party in my pants. Want to cum?
Don't be silly. I wouldn't want to disrupt your fun.

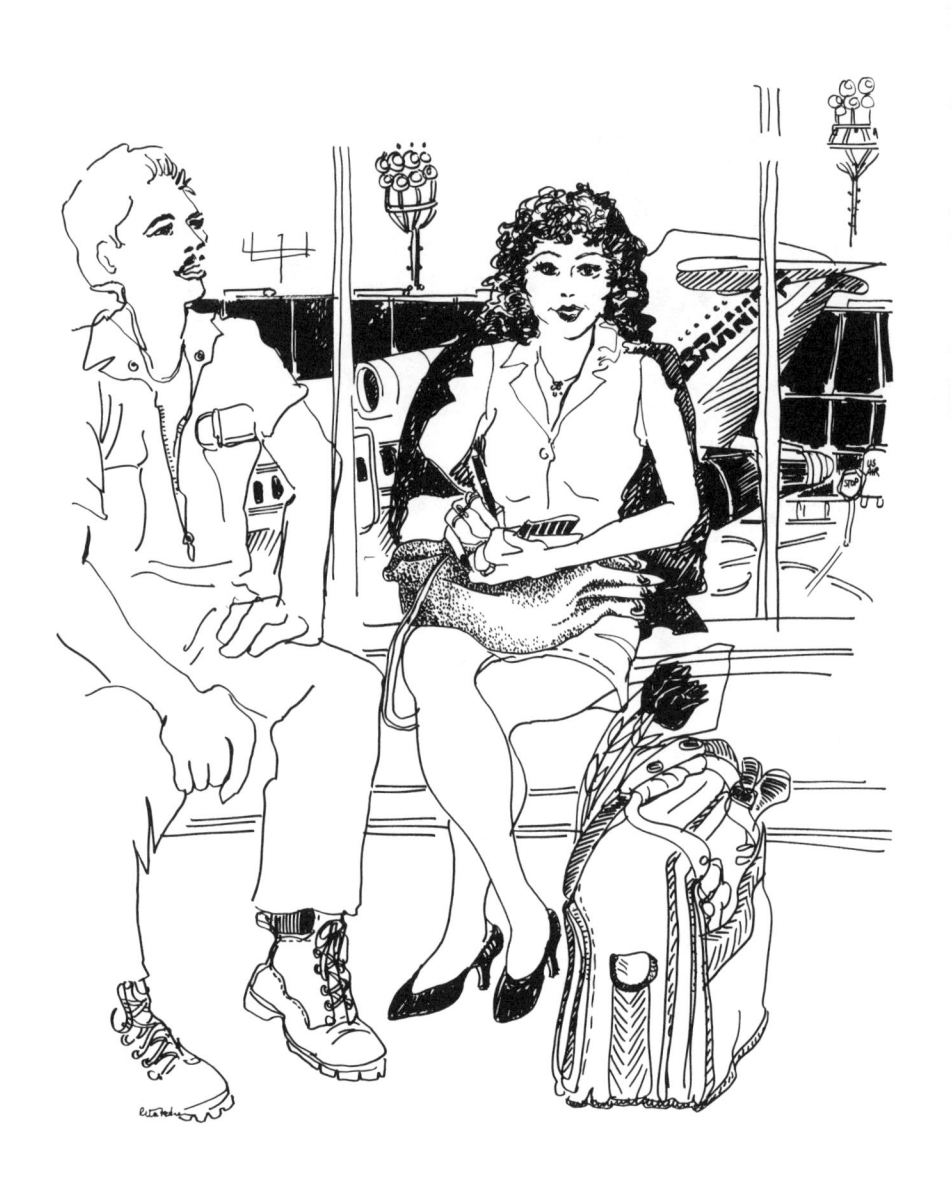

He: Hey, baby, why don't you come fly with me?
She: Have you got an extra white bag?

AIR LINES

Hi there, sweety; how about joining me for a cocktail before take-off?
> *No thanks. I'm taking off right now!*

Sometimes flying makes me full of lust and lightheadedness....
> *That's not all it makes you full of!*

Why don't you tune into my channel, honey-cups?
> *No thank you, I've tuned out for the rest of the flight.*

Please comfort me. I'm simply petrified of flying alone!
> *Gee, I'm sorry, I didn't know they allowed ancient trees on planes.*

I hate how my shorts creep on these long flights, don't you?
> *No, I hate sitting next to short creeps like you.*

Hey, baby, why don't you come fly with me?
> *Have you got an extra white bag?*

FRATERNITY LINES

Tonight is your lucky night! You met me at this fraternity party.
Tonight is your unlucky night. I hold a black belt in karate.

Would you like to be a Little Sister?
No thanks, I'm the oldest of four.

I've never been upstairs in a sorority.
It's just like the downstairs, only harder to get to.

My frat house is having a party, and my room is going to be crowded, so can I sleep over at your house?
Gee, I'd rather go to the party.

I have better booze upstairs in my room. Would you like to come up for a drink?
Is that why you serve the cheap stuff downstairs?

I always thought that sorority girls were such snobs, but you're so warm and friendly.
We are, but if you don't remove your hand from my ass, I'll make sure that you'll never think again!

Have you had a house tour?
You've seen one, you've seen them all.

You know that rumor about the ancient Greeks isn't true of us modern Greeks.
Too bad. They were great philosophers and thinking men.

WAY-OUT LINES

How about you and me experiencing the outer limits together?
That's right; I'm out of your limits.

I want to blast my rocket through your solar system.
Sorry, I'm having my eclipse.

When I look at you I see a sophisticated product of high-tech engineering . . . I'll bet you can really perform.
Fine equipment is useless in the hands of amateurs.

Hi! I'm a practicing heterosexual. Would you like to come and practice with me?
No thanks, I don't need practice.

Hey, baby, let me take you to paradise.
The travel agent doesn't open until 10:00 A.M.

You must be a Libra. You're so well-balanced and perfectly proportioned.
Wrong. I'm a Virgo—the virgin—and I'm planning on staying that way for a while.

BEACH LINES

That towel looks big enough for both of us.
> *Actually, it's only big enough for my boyfriend and me.*

Want to come upstairs and compare tan lines?
> *No, I lie on nude beaches.*

How long have you been down here?
> *Obviously too long.*

Your hotel or mine?
> *Sorry, I'm staying at my grandmother's.*

You're sunbathing in the exact same spot where I fell in love for the first time.
> *Obviously it's an unlucky spot.*

Wow, you have the most gorgeous, penetrating blue eyes I've ever seen.
> *You must have x-ray vision to be able to see through my sunglasses.*

Hey, gorgeous, how about giving me a ride to the beach?
> *No thanks. Looks like you could use the exercise.*

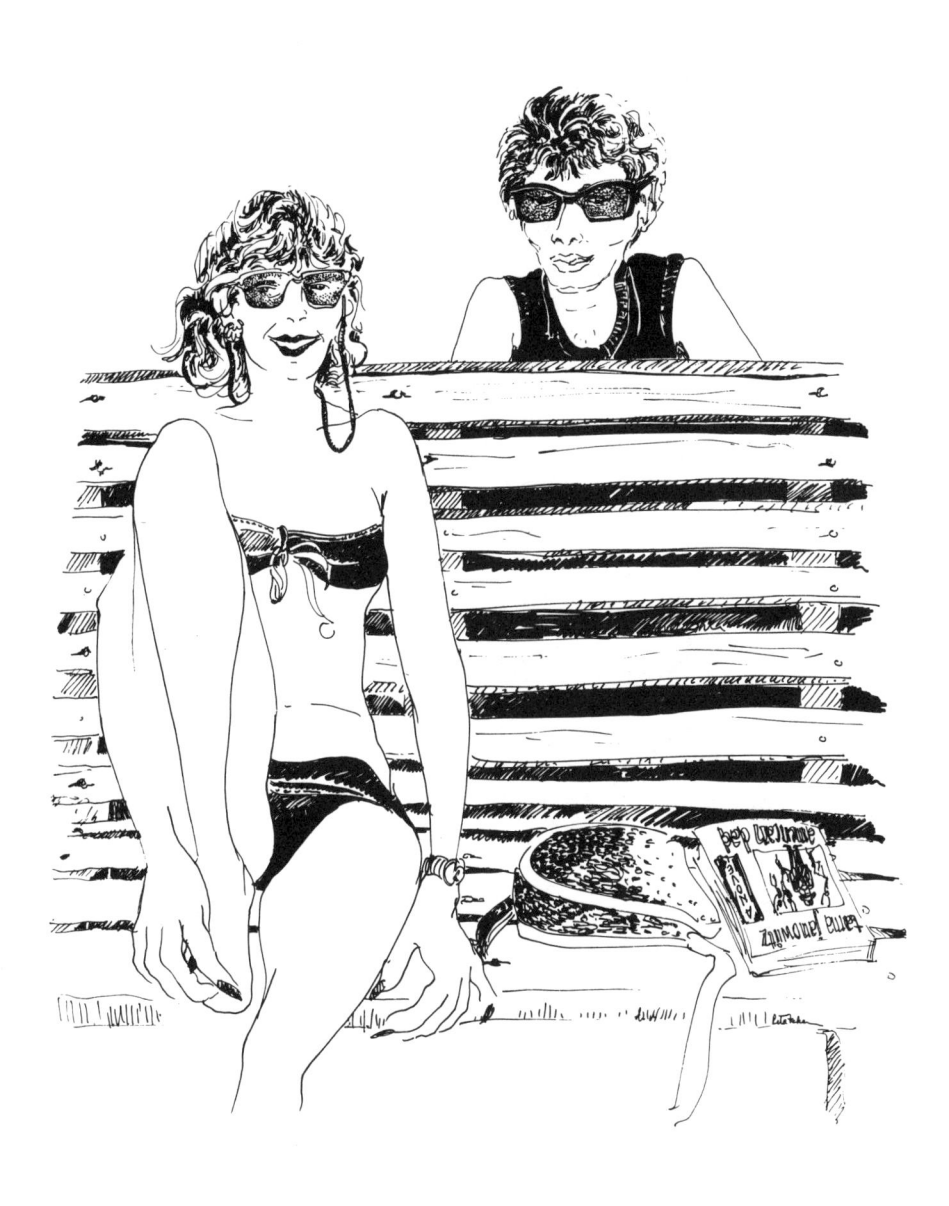

He: Wow, you have the most gorgeous, penetrating blue eyes I've ever seen.
She: You must have x-ray vision to be able to see through my sunglasses.

CAR
LINES

Want me to check your oil?
> *No thanks. If I get filled, I get zits.*

Would you like me to charge your battery?
> *You do not have enough electricity!*

Would you like me to fill your tank?
> *No thanks. I take premium.*

Would you like me to gap your plugs?
> *No, I already had a tune-up.*

Can I shine your headlights?
> *I doubt it. I have to be turned on to make them shine!*

I want to give you a free body job.
> *I will bring my car in tomorrow!*
> or
> *What is wrong with it the way it is?*
> or
> *No, that would require a skilled craftsman.*

I'd like to put my motor in drive.
> *Well, back off, because I'm in reverse.*

I'm revving up my engine.
> *Too bad, my batteries are dead.*

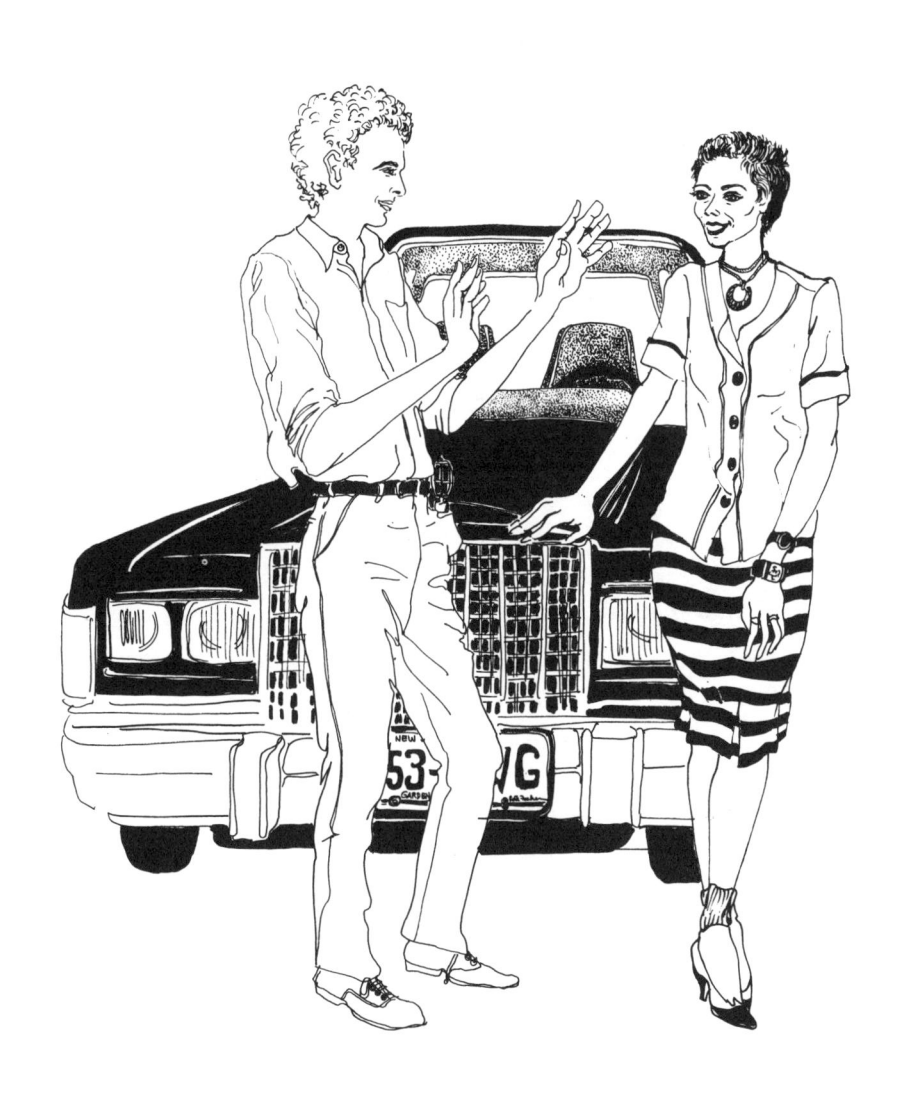

He: I want to give you a free body job.
She: No, that would require a *skilled* craftsman.

Let me make your motor hum.
>   *No thanks, I had a tune-up last week.*
>   or
>   *I didn't know that you are a mechanic.*

I'll keep you warm.
>   *I think I'd rather freeze.*

This car is too small. Want to go look for a van?
>   *No, I do my best controlling during the daytime.*

Want to go for a ride?
>   *I don't think so; I get bored easily.*

Hey, baby, pump me.
>   *This is a self-service station. Pump your own.*

Can you check under my hood?
>   *Wait a minute, I'll close the station.*

MEDICAL LINES

I've taken anatomy. I know where all your *erogenous* zones are.
Sorry, I think you've been given some erroneous *information.*

I'm a pre-med major. That means I'm a smooth *operator.*
I hope you have malpractice insurance, because you just blew this operation.

C'mon, sex is a natural biological function.
Not with you it isn't.

If fertilization does occur, termination of zygote formation is a simple procedure.
For you maybe, but not for me!

I can't help myself. Wanting to have sex with you is an instinctive urge.
My instinct tells me I should leave.

When you're near, my hormone levels begin to rise, muscular tension increases, my heart rate increases, my blood pressures increases, and vasocongestion occurs in my pelvic area. I can't control myself.
I bet you say that to all the girls.

Want to play doctor?
Why, are you sick?

Have you had a shot before?
No, but I don't want to be pricked.

BAR LINES

Wow! I don't meet too many people who drink _____ too.

Do you want to come back to my apartment and catch a good movie on my new VCR after this bar closes?

I hate crowds, don't you?
> *Yes, and you're crowding me.*

Let's go home and hop each other's bones.
> *If only I'd known; I already fed mine to the dog.*

Let's go home and stain my sheets.
> *I'd rather refinish a cabinet.*

Let's take a ride on the wild side.
> *No thanks, I never take sides.*

Let's go back to my place and get naked.
> *[Look at him/her from head to toe.] Nah, I don't think so.*
>   or
> *O.K., I'm ready for a good laugh.*

Want to check out my waterbed?
> *Why, is that out of control, too?*
>   or
> *Why, are you going away for the weekend?*

Let's get horizontal.
> *No, I'd rather be vertical.*

LANDSCAPING LINES

Did you know that landscapers plant it deeper?
Deeper than what?

Did you know we do it in the dirt?
Well forget it, I keep my house clean!

Would you like to plant my tree?
No, I think it already died!

Would you like me to trim your bush?
No, I take care of all my own maintenance.

Do you want to help me plant my bulbs?
Let's wait until they mature!

Would you like me to fill your hole?
I doubt if you have enough clean fill.

I would like to water your flower.
It is on an automatic watering system.

Do you want me to fertilize your flower?
No, I don't want fruit!

COLLEGE LINES

Aren't you in my English class?
  No hablo ingles.

Aren't you in my anthropology class?
  No, but I see you've learned primitive behavior.

Law student: How'd you like to see my briefs?

Film major: Let's cut to my place.

Geology: Come home with me, and I'll show you my rock collection.

Business: I'd like to check your accounts.

Economics: I know my demand. How is your supply?

Engineer: Do you want to blow the big one?
  Sure, if I can find it.

Geography: I want to explore you.
  Why don't you explore the room instead—maybe you'll find the door.

Philosophy: At this stage of our relationship, it's the logical thing to do.
  Don't you think it would be more logical if we wait until I'm ready?

Psychology: I'm interested in your body *and* your mind.
That's funny—I'm not interested in your body or *your mind.*

Religion: What's the matter? God won't punish you!
No, but I will!

Sociology: Everybody's doing it.
I'm not.

Forestry: I'm not really a "stumpy" if you know what I mean.
You will be if you don't cool it.

Television: I'm sure you'll give me a high rating.
Wrong—you've just been canceled.

Astronomy: I know that kiss made you see stars—how would you like to see a super-nova?
Why don't you blast-off!

Greek literature: The Gods used to do it all the time.
And look where it got them.

Physical education: It's not healthy to get excited and not follow through with it.
Then leave—that should curb your excitement.

Drama: When we're done, you'll want to give me an Oscar.
I'd rather try out someone else for the part.

OUT-OF-THE-ORDINARY LINES

I promise this isn't a line.

Haven't I seen you in my wet dreams?

Do me, baby, like I've never been done before.

I'm so juicy.

You light my fire.

Give it to me—give me some more of that funky stuff.

I'll be your freakazoid; all you have to do is wind me up.

If I told you I was a turtle, would you help me out of my shell?

I can tell you've been dying to meet me.

Can I have a bite?

I really like those pants you're wearing. Can I talk you out of them?

What does your dog do on its day off?

Blue eyes are my favorite.
   Mine too; yours are brown.

Don't you like men?
> *Why, are you writing a book?*

Yeah.
> *Well, make it a mystery.*

If you give me a backrub, I'll give you one too.
> *Sorry, you rub me the wrong way.*

Ju tu adore. That's French.
> *Vie Doncha—Fuck off. That's Russian.*

This is my first night out. I'm not what you think.
> *I'm glad, for a moment I thought you were a hooker.*

You can't get what I have anywhere else.
> *Really? I didn't know herpes was so scarce in this town.*

We really love each other, so why should we wait?
> *It's because we love each other that we* can *wait.*

Spending all that money on dinner, don't I get something?
> *Yeah, indigestion.*

What's a nice girl like you doing in a place like this?
> *Looking for an exit.*

Hey, let's blow this place and go back to my apartment for some real action.
> *If the party is only in your pants, I don't want to come.*

Is it true that blondes have the most fun?
> *Yes, too bad you aren't a blonde.*

I think you're really sexy.
> *Thanks, my boyfriend thinks so too.*

You're short. Can I pick you up?
> *No, I like the view down here.*

Hey, sweetheart. I know you haven't heard from me in a while...
> *If I wanted to hear from an asshole, I would have farted.*

I've got something you've always wanted from a guy.
  A diamond ring?

What has thirty-eight teeth and holds back the incredible hulk?
  What?
My zipper.
  I hope it holds long enough for me to get out of here.

You have one big middle-class hangup.
  It's you that has the hangup—one big hard on.

I feel like an animal when I'm around you.
  Should I spread some newspaper?

Trust me.
  Yes, I will, but need I go to bed with you to trust you?

I have enough cash to make you eternally happy!
  Well, let me have it and leave me forever alone!

Does that necklace mean you're spoken for?
  No, I speak for myself.

I'm ape for your shape.
  Thanks, but I don't monkey around.

Has anyone ever told you that you have beautiful calves?
  No, but I've been called a mighty mean heifer before.

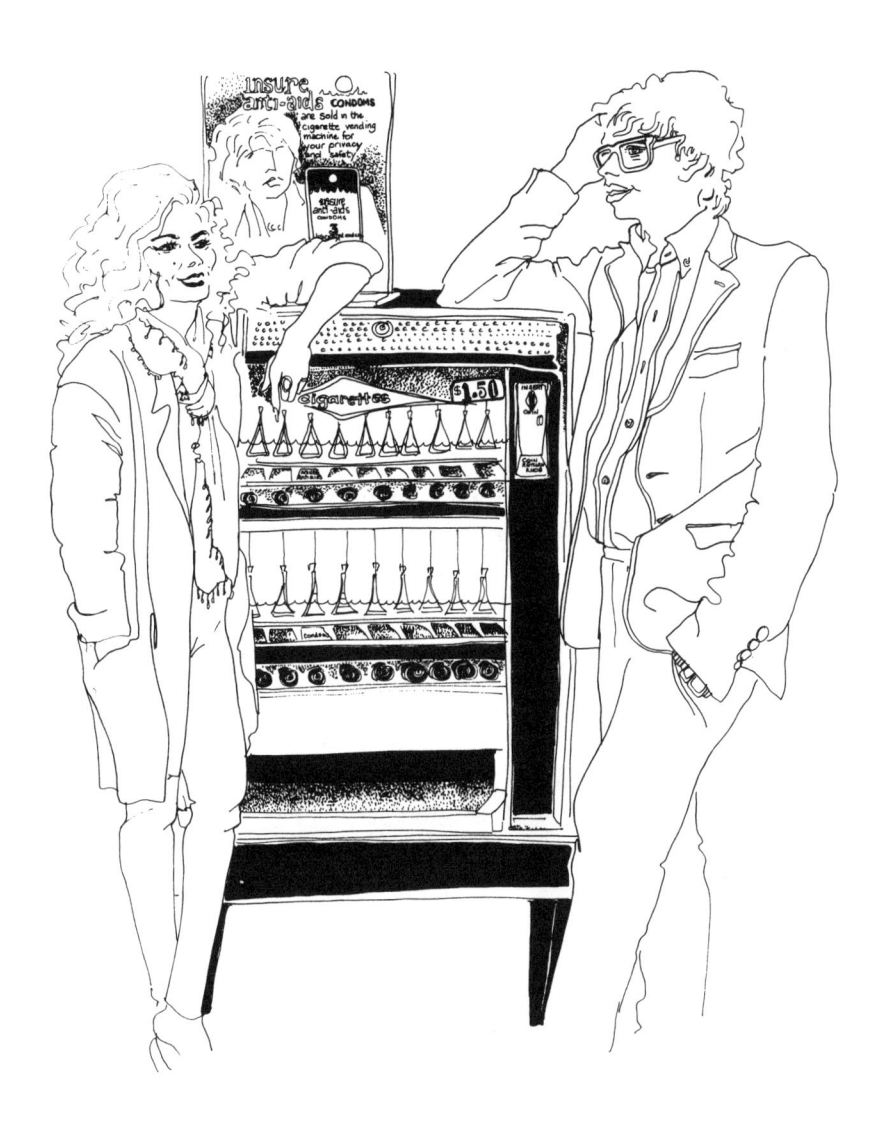

He: It will ruin the mood if I wear a condom.
She: It will ruin more than the mood if I get pregnant.

BIRTH CONTROL LINES

Birth control isn't romantic.

It's not natural for me to wear a condom.
It's not natural for me to have an abortion either.

It will ruin the mood if I wear a condom.
It will ruin more than the mood if I get pregnant.

It's too embarrassing to buy condoms.
But it's only a minor inconvenience to have a baby?

If you get pregnant, I'll give you the money to have an abortion.
For a fraction of what an abortion costs, you can buy a condom.

If you get pregnant, I'll take care of you.
You can start caring for me now by wearing a condom.

Wearing a condom is like taking a shower with a raincoat on.
Maybe that's what you need—a cold shower.

Birth control pills are hazardous to your health.
Pregnancy is more of a stress.

Why don't we play doctor?
After we play planned parenthood.

FATE AND INTELLECTUAL LINES

You have an interesting perspective of Plato (economics, poetry, genetics, etc.). I would love to have you expound further on the subject.

You are so different from the other students; I feel so comfortable with you.

You're a rare combination of beauty and intellect. I would like to get to know you.

I would love to discuss *Paradise Lost* with you in a quiet place.

It is destiny. Fate. You were meant to be with me tonight.
You don't have much vision if you are only concerned with tonight.

I am a hedonist. I seek pleasure from you.
Too bad; I'm into S and M.

Don't you feel that this is the beginning of something meaningful?
No, try the end of something meaningless.

NEW RESPONSES TO OLD LINES

Hey, baby, do you want to get lucky?
Why, are you a fairy?
   or
Thanks, but I'll keep looking for four-leaf clovers.

We should really be honest with each other.
If I were any more honest, I'd call the police.

Want to make a few memories?
Yeah, but I'd prefer to make some I won't have to try to forget later.

Let's do a little pleasin' instead of teasin'.
If I thought you could please, I wouldn't tease.

Want to come in for a nightcap?
Only if it goes with a nightshirt.
   or
I only drink fresh palm wine at night.

This is the chance of a lifetime.
I guess I'm unlucky.

I'd like to share some time with you.
You can share all the time you want, but not any space.

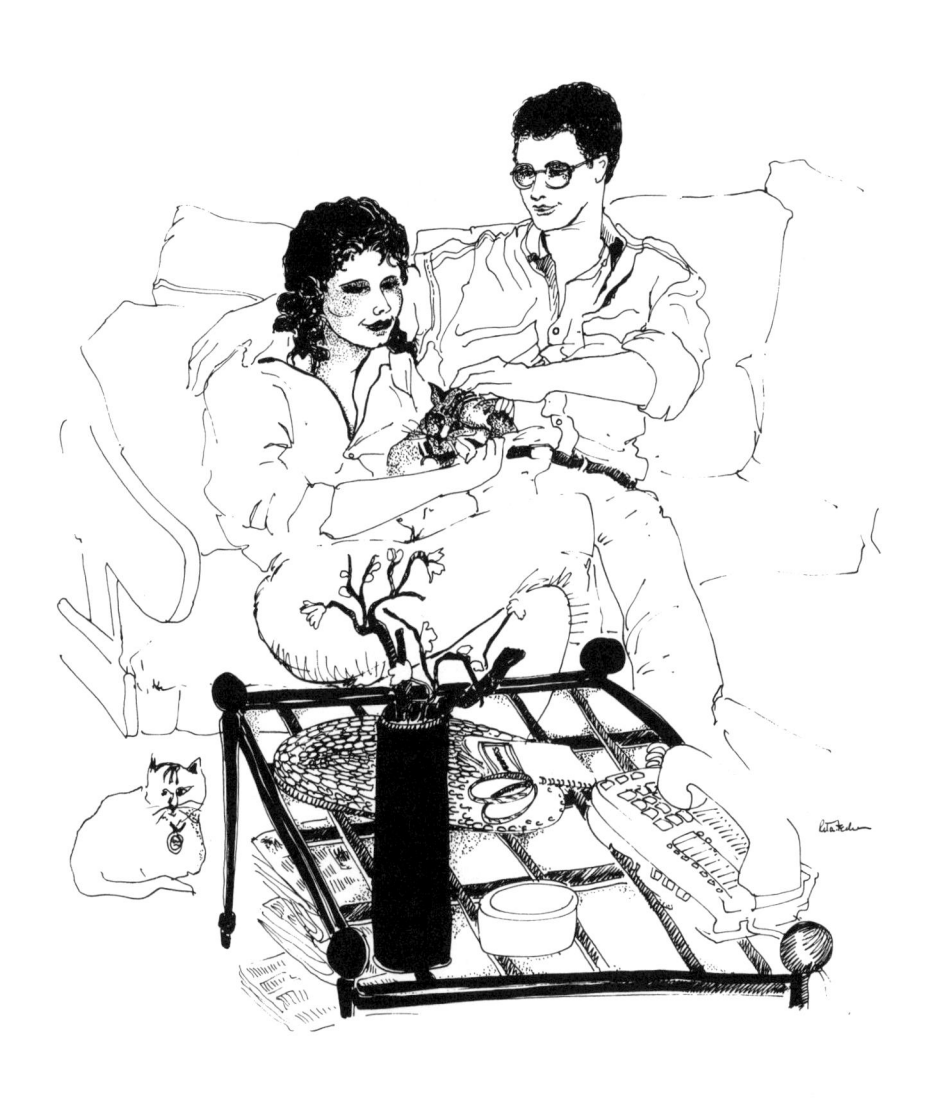

He: Want to make a few memories?
She: Yeah, but I'd prefer to make some I won't have to try to forget later.

You look bored.
>   *No, but I have the feeling that I will be soon.*

I just want to be close to you.
>   *That's a little too close for comfort.*

You're not a little girl anymore. You can make your own decisions.
>   *Then my decision is no.*

Do you have the time?
>   *Not for you.*

They're playing our song.
>   *Sorry, but you're way off key.*

I've been watching you all night; I just couldn't keep my eyes off you!
>   *I've been watching you too, and I know all your moves.*

COWBOY LINES

I swear, y'all must be the yellow rose of Texas.
And you're the thorn in my side.

I would love to saddle-up on y'all.
You must be in the wrong place. I believe the corral is farther down the road.

Yee-ha! You are a fighter—I love bustin' bronco.
You'd better leave me alone, or I'll bust your bronco.

It's no use fighting, babe. Don't y'all know that cowboys always get their man?
If it's a man that you are looking for, I think you'd better open your eyes and look elsewhere.

Southern nights are for lovers.
My southern nights are for sleeping . . . alone.

You're one lucky Yankee. I've decided to take you on a tour of the nicest sights in Texas.
The best sights are those where I don't see you.

I can think of better ways for you to use that pretty little tongue than playing hard to get.
You are not getting it.

COMPUTER LINES

Would you like to interface?

You have terrific software.

You can insert my floppy disc anytime.

Let's switch to the binary mode.

Do you think I could teach you the Basics?
> *You probably could; it's just that I'm not into computer programming.*

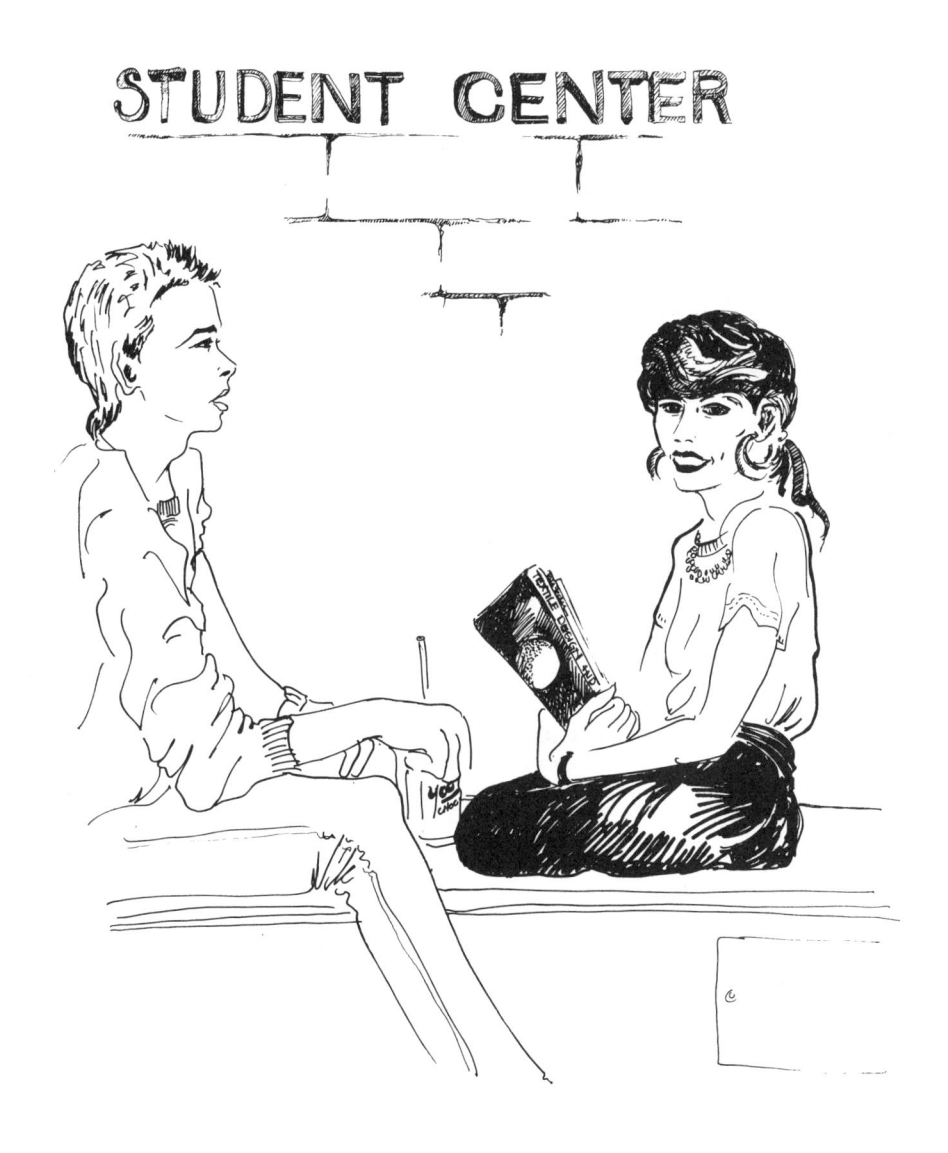

He: Do you think I could teach you the Basics?
She: You probably could; it's just that I'm not into computer programming.

HISPANIC-AMERICAN LINES

I've always wanted a nice dark-skinned girl like you.

Please, mama, give me a kiss.

I want to show you a good time.

I know what you need, and I'm going to give it to you.

I'm going to love you like you've never been loved before.

I want to feel all of your warmth, pretty lady.

Put your hand on me, sweetheart. Make me drunk with your love.

Come enjoy yourself now, because this time will never come again.

If you cook the way you walk, I'll marry you.

LINES USED BY JEWS

Want to play put the lox in the bagel?

Want to cream my cheese?

You remind me of my mother. I love my mother. Are you interested?
Why settle for second-best?

You know, Jewish guys are stereotyped as having small penises, but I'm the exception. Do you want proof?
You know, Jewish girls are stereotyped as being easy to take to bed, but I'm the exception to that rule. Need any more proof?

My rabbi says it's O.K. to have premarital sex.
Then go have sex with your rabbi.

Want to taste my matza balls?
No thanks. My Grandmother makes great ones.

My parents only let me go out with nice Jewish girls like you.
Who said I'm a nice Jewish girl?

GAY
LINES

How long have you been out of the closet?
I was out, but now I think I'll go back in.

Hey, butch, I bet I can please you like no man ever has.
Oh really. Does that mean you're paying for dinner?

Do you think you could handle both of us?
No, it's all I can do to handle one asshole at a time.

Hi, I'm ten inches and horny and I like what you got.
Sorry, I choke on five.

LINES USED BY BLACKS

Hey, baby—my name is Kevin; take my hand and I'll lead you to heaven.

Virgins are my specialty—over fifty million served.

If I go on to someone else, don't blame me.

A man can't live without sex.

It would prove our love for each other.

Birth control isn't romantic.

Why do you keep on teasing me, when you won't give it up?

Just let's be natural.

You are fine as wine.

You make me burn with desire.

You are my everything, honey sugar. If I can't hug and make love to you I'll go crazy.

I won't tell a soul, baby. No one has to know—if you want to be totally discrete.

Foxy mama, let me put some good lovin' on you.

Get with it; this is the '80s.
Get with it. You ain't getting none from me.

If you come out with me, I'll treat you to anything you want. How about it, baby?
Oh yeah—you'll treat me to a baby!

COSMIC, CELESTIAL, AND STAR WARS LINES

Do you want to come on a cosmic trip with me?

We're orbiting the same sphere. Why not convene for a thorough strategy check?

The impact will be intense, but after that it's celestial.

Let me experience you in 3-D, baby!

Hook up to my terminal—the output sensations are terrific.

Video stimulation is fantastic, but I need tactile to make it *real*.

The harmonic distortion of our relationship would be eliminated if you'd just cooperate.

This planet is so cold and inhuman. Please help fill the void.

You mesmerize my entire source.

Utopia is here and now, baby. Let's experience it as one "organism."

I've got a missile ready to deploy—and you'd make a perfect launch site.

The logistics are simple. You remove your zipsuit, and I'll let my transmitter probe your depth.

We could formulate a perfect concept of ecstasy.

Tonight I'm programmed for viceral activities—so don't be an alien.

Are you trying to sabotage my neural synapse by denying me?

Our magnetic fields show mutual attraction. Let's join forces.

I'm in suspended animation without you.

There's no gravity where I can take you.

Think of it this way: It'd be a fusion of two beautiful elements.

Want to relocate to my "launch pad"?

Genetic engineering couldn't have made a more perfect specimen than you.

My system's energized for some dynamic interaction.

Let's synthesize body chemistries.

How about entering a time warp together and doing some body exploration?

Freud was last century; my only hang-up is your archaic attitude toward humanoid sex.

You don't have anything to worry about—I'll break the circuit just before emitting the Milky Way.

I've got a laser to put you into orbit!

You're eclipsing my excited state with your ancient viewpoint about sex.

But I love you—nucleus, matrix, and brain waves.

My solar warmth will penetrate you gently.

Think of it as a spontaneous energy exchange.

Your static attitude could cause future mutations.

This is a pluralistic society; you really have limited scope.

We could transcend the galaxy together.

My love for you supercedes an atomic explosion.

Schematically, we'd make an ideal merger.

Forming an alliance will illuminate a new theory about sex for you.

Hey, I detect heavy vibes radiating from your direction. Let's see how much kinetic energy we can create.

Let's get our frequencies together for some high voltage fun.

The medium is our bodies; the message is infrared!

I'd just like to monitor your pubic area with my instrument.

Our relationship would be much more systematized with sex.

I seem to be short-circuited. Can I recharge on you?

My scientific rationalization occasionally gives way to earthy impulses.
What's so cosmic about that?

VIDEO GAME LINES

Did you know that video games are very sexual? Certain games girls are attracted to, and certain games guys enjoy. Games that shoot out things, like Asteroids, guys like; games that eat up and take things in are popular with women, like Pac-Man.
Do you like to shoot things out?
Yeah.
Good. I enjoy watching things shoot out. The door's over there.

Pac-Man is very good for eye-hand coordination. I'm sure you have good hands.
Too bad you won't find out.

My joystick works better than that machine's.
It won't score around here.

How about coming over and playing with my joystick?
No thanks. I have Intellivision at home.

You wanna play a game?
Depends. What does the winner get?
Wait and find out.
I don't like waiting.

Do you play much?
You'll never find out.

I have Atari at home. Do you want to come over? We can play all night long, and it's free.
Well, I'm not free.

MISCELLANEOUS LINES

MARRIED LINES

Does that ring mean you are spoken for?
No, I speak for myself.

You have a hang-up about married men!
No, it's you who as a hang-up about being married.

DREAM LINES

I dream about making love to you.
Keep dreaming.

I dream about making it with you every night and get such an exciting feeling all over my body. Would you like to make it with me?
No thank you, stick with your dreams, it sounds like you're already having a good time.

I dreamed of you last night.
Did you get to the part where I reject you?

DOWN ON THE FARM LINES

Want to take a little roll in the hay?
No, I don't like crumbs (human or edible) in bed.

Let's make the feathers fly.
> *No, chickens and turkeys don't mix.*

SMELL LINES

You smell great. What's that you have on?
> *Raid, so bug off, pest!*

You smell so sensuous. What kind of perfume are you wearing?
> *Right Guard.*

Do you want to have some fun? Get my drift?
> *The only drift I get from you is your body odor.*

INTERNATIONAL LINES

CANADIAN LINES

If you really love me, why don't you prove it?

If you are really Canadian, show me your beaver!

Let me plough your field.

Come on, these are the eighties.

Excuse me, I am looking for an orgasm. I was wondering if you could help me.

Do you want to exchange gum?

I'd like to butter your muffin.

You're very beautiful. I can't help myself.

If I told you that you have a beautiful body, would you hold it against me?

Tickle my tonsils.

Relax.

I've had sex before, but I've never made love. I want you to be the first girl I *make love* to.

Nobody has to know.

If you are a man, prove it.

Hey, babe, do you want to be like John Wayne and get back in the saddle?

Don't worry; sixteen is old enough. You are not a baby any more.

You teased me. It's not fair if you don't follow through.

Put out or get out.

If you'd have sex with me, you'd make me the happiest guy in the world.

Hello, babe. Want some special candy?

Give me a break.

I don't think you like me any more.

Want to go watch the submarine races?

Are the buttons on those pants edible?

I can see myself getting married to someone like you.

I'll pull out in time.

Hey, baby, take a walk on my wild side.

Don't think I'm coming on to you or anything.

You and I are made for each other.

You know, you look like this guy at my old school.

Don't worry, I'll respect you in the morning.

Why don't you trust me when I've told you I love you?

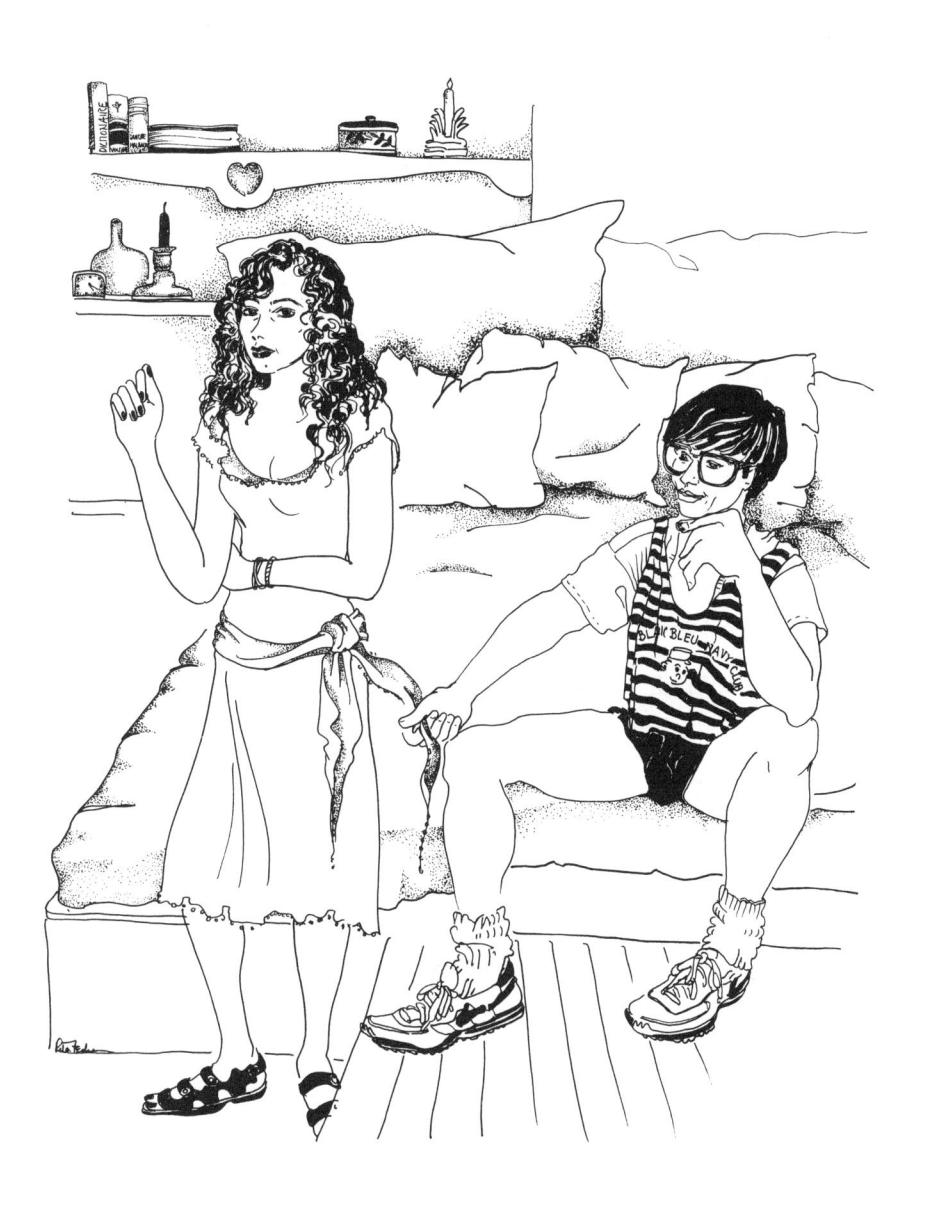

He: Everybody does it.
She: So you won't have any trouble finding someone else to do it with.

Hey, baby, do you want to be my sledgehammer?

I'm overworked, oversexed, and over here.

Why can't you just calm down and do it?

I'm warm for your form.

I'm trying to be your friend and help you through your fears.

You drive me wild with desire.
> *But my desire is to drive you home.*

Everybody does it.
> *I'm not everybody.*
>   or
> *So you won't have any trouble finding someone else to do it with.*

If you don't, I'll break up with you.
> *If you're willing to make that kind of a threat, you'll probably break up with me right after we do it, so what's the point?*

A guy could get sick or die if he stopped.
> *I'll be at your funeral.*

Want to warm up your fingers?
> *That's O.K. I'm wearing gloves.*

Hi, have we met before?
> *Have we?*

If it's your first time, you can't get pregnant.
> *Of course you can. Everybody knows that.*

Where have you been all my life?
> *Hiding from you.*

But I'll get blue balls.
> *If you don't get out of here, they'll be black and blue.*

BRITISH LINES

We love each other. Let's fulfill this love.

If you're not a virgin anymore, one more time won't hurt.

Soon you'll be the only virgin left.

I'll show you how to come properly.

You're tense. If you let me put it in, it will relax you.

I'm not going to do anything to you.

It's natural for two people like us.

If you understand me . . .

Be with it!

You're a professional virgin.

I've always wanted to be loved like this.

I would like to lose my virginity to you, Sugar.

It will be okay because I love you.

You're a dumb kid to keep saying no; look what you're missing!

Let's be together, warm and comfortable somewhere, *you* know.

I've had the operation!!

You're grown up now; it's your body. You don't have to do what Mummy says.

Haven't you ever had sex with a black boy before? Then you're missing something.

Why should you be so selfish with yourself? I'm so lonely and I need you so much. Please be a little bit generous.

It's healthier to do it.

You might as well—it'll only take a minute.

Don't be a prickteaser.

Everything's been really getting me down lately.

Let's just say you and I wanted to have sex . . .

Do you think you can last the distance?

I fancy you.

There is a great view of the city from my flat.

You can't get pregnant if you sneeze afterwards.

You can't get pregnant if you jump up and down or go dancing afterwards.

You can't get pregnant if you do it more than three times in one night.

You can't get pregnant if you go to the lavatory afterwards.

Can I ring you?
Why don't you wring your neck?

IRISH LINES

I'd love to bury my head in your clover patch.

(After a pinch . . .) My, what rosey cheeks ya have, darlin'.

(After a dance . . .) Would ya like to go to my place and see how we do a different type of jig?

A little leprechaun told me you were starin' my way and thought it'd be a good idea for me to try and strike up a conversation with ya.

GERMAN LINES

If you really love me, you can easily prove it to me with sex.

Would you like to have a really good time?

If you love me, then you'll let me make love to you. Love and sex go together.

Hey, sweety, let's get it on!
    I'd rather get out!

Where have you been all my life?
    Nicely hidden, and now I'd like to disappear again, if you please.

Your eyes tell me a story I have never known.
    And will never be known to you!

You are the sexiest man in this place!
    Thanks, but no thanks.

It is so hot in here! Come to the garden with me to cool off.
    No! I can't imagine you'd let things cool off out there.

I know a lovely spot nearby. Will you take a walk with me?
    What! Walk? Never. No thanks!

Will you come up for a nightcap?
    Of course not! You already smell like a brewery.

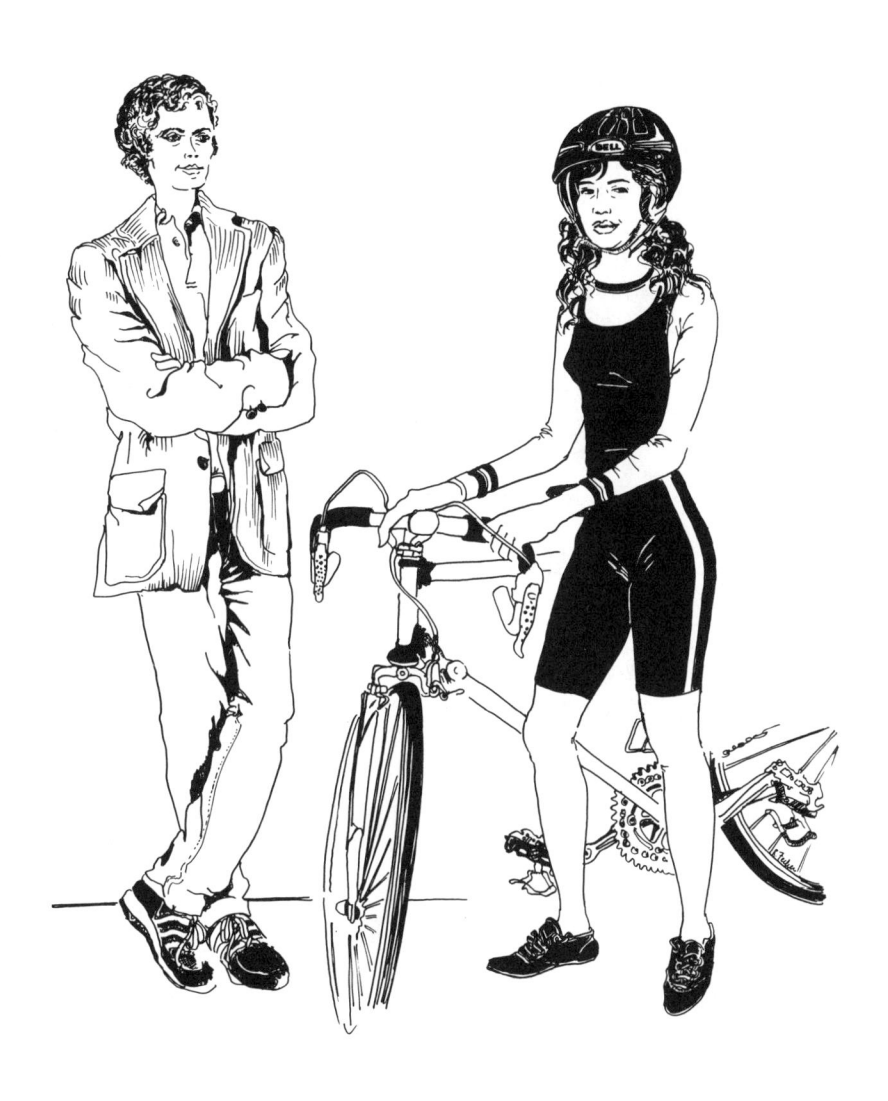

He: Where have you been all my life?
She: Nicely hidden, and now I'd like to disappear again, if you please.

I need passion. I mean deep passion.
> *What you need is a shrink. I mean a good one!*

The night is like blue velvet!
> *You sound like you are drunk.*

Our souls have the same vibes.
> *Too bad the vibes are out of phase, babe!*

Just one little kiss?
> *Save it! Maybe someday you can afford a big kiss ... for someone else.*

You have a very beautiful face!
> *Look, that's nice, but there's more to my person than just a beautiful face. If you fail to realize that, it pisses me off, so why don't you just piss off!*

You are a special person to me.
> *Yes. I'm so special that I don't want anything to do with you!*

I'd like to know more about you.
> *You need to know only one thing and that is that you make me sick.*

How would you like to come out and play?
> *How would you like to fuck off and die?*

NORWEGIAN LINES

Do you want to make love to me?

Your eyes are like violets, not because they are so blue, but because they sit on a stem (stick out).

Your eyes are like the ocean, not because they are so blue, but because they are so watery.

Don't worry, I will be very careful.

Do you want to come and hear my new album?
   No thanks, I've heard it before.

DUTCH LINES

If you really love me, you'll have sex with me.

Do you have the time?

Have I seen you on television recently?

May I offer you a drink?

Are you related to ―――――― ?

You look like someone I know.

Do you have a cigarette?

Do you want to sail with me?

If you say *A* then you have to say *B*.
  I didn't say A *at all.*

Haven't I seen you before?
  Not that I can remember.

UKRANIAN
LINES

You would if you loved me.

I want you and need you right now!

My dark eyes meet yours.

My heart belongs to you.

I like to watch you get water; also I love you like the wind loves the moon and the stars.

GREEK LINES

If you really love me, you'll have sex with me.

I could beat around the bush a little more and we could do a lot of role playing, but I find you very attractive and I'd really like to make love to you.

You are backward.

You are narrow-minded.

Everybody is doing it. Why don't you try?

You don't accept me because you don't love me.

That's why I prefer the foreign girls; they are progressive and they don't mind doing it.

It's about time that you changed your mind about the virtues of virginity.

If you don't want to do it, I'll find another girl who will.

Do you want to dance?
    No.
Then I guess a night in the sack is out of the question?

Do you want to get lucky tonight?
    O.K., let's go to Parnitha [a casino]!

TURKISH LINES

Could I offer you a drink?
Yes, if you feel like it.

Would you like to come to my house? We can have a nice time.
Thanks for the drink, but I'd prefer spending the night with another guy!

FRENCH LINES

French is such a beautiful language; I could listen to you speak it all night.

Is it true what they say about French women?

Have you ever seen the Eiffel Tower at midnight?

Can you direct me to the nearest hotel?

What's a nice girl like you doing in a place like this?

Aren't you a dancer at the Moulin Rouge [famous strip joint in Paris]?

What do you think about Mitterand's foreign policy?

Do you want to make love to me?

No one stays a virgin for very long.

What are you doing tonight?

Are you French [even when they know you're not]?

How about a bit of coq au vin?

Do you want to go to bed with me tonight?
    No, if I went to bed with you, all I'd do is sleep.

You have a body made for love.
> *I know, and I'm still waiting for the right person to share it with.*

Is there a place where we can go alone?
> *No, but I know a place where you can go alone.*

SPANISH AND SOME SOUTH AMERICAN LINES

If the merchandise is for sale, I'll buy the whole store.

I have a table for two, but one of the seats is empty.

Can I ride my tongue down your highway?

Do you have a light?
> *If I do, it may take a while to warm up.*

You are harder than the street and better tasting than the Lipton soups.
> *Your compliments would even shock a whore.*

I would eat you even with your clothing on; it doesn't matter if I end up shitting rags for a month.
> *You probably will when you see what I'm wearing underneath this rag.*

So many curves and I'm without brakes.
> *Then I'll apply my own.*

So much meat and I'm on a diet.
> *Then it would be a good idea to go see Weight Watchers.*

You are good, honey.
>   *You'll never get close enough to find out.*

What a pan, and here I am with my eggs [testicles] raw.
>   *Check your temperature; from the looks of things you're hotter than you think.*

Aren't you in my class?
>   *You don't have class.*

Why don't you go to the Casbah?
>   *Why don't you go—away?*

Where are you, my love?
>   *I'm not your love.*

Hi, how are you?
>   *I was fine until I saw you!*

Do you want to go out for some fresh air?
>   *The air was fresh in here until you came over!*

Your ass looks cute when you dance. I bet it looks better in bed!
>   *You wouldn't like it, it has pimples on it!*

Hi, do you come here often?
>   *I did, but I won't anymore!*

I want you to have my baby.
>   *I would never have the son of Frankenstein!*

Listen, love, do you want to spend some time with a sweet loving man?
>   *Well, when I find one, I'll be sure to treat him right.*

You know that I can satisfy your every desire.
>   *If that's the case, then change me into cold ice.*

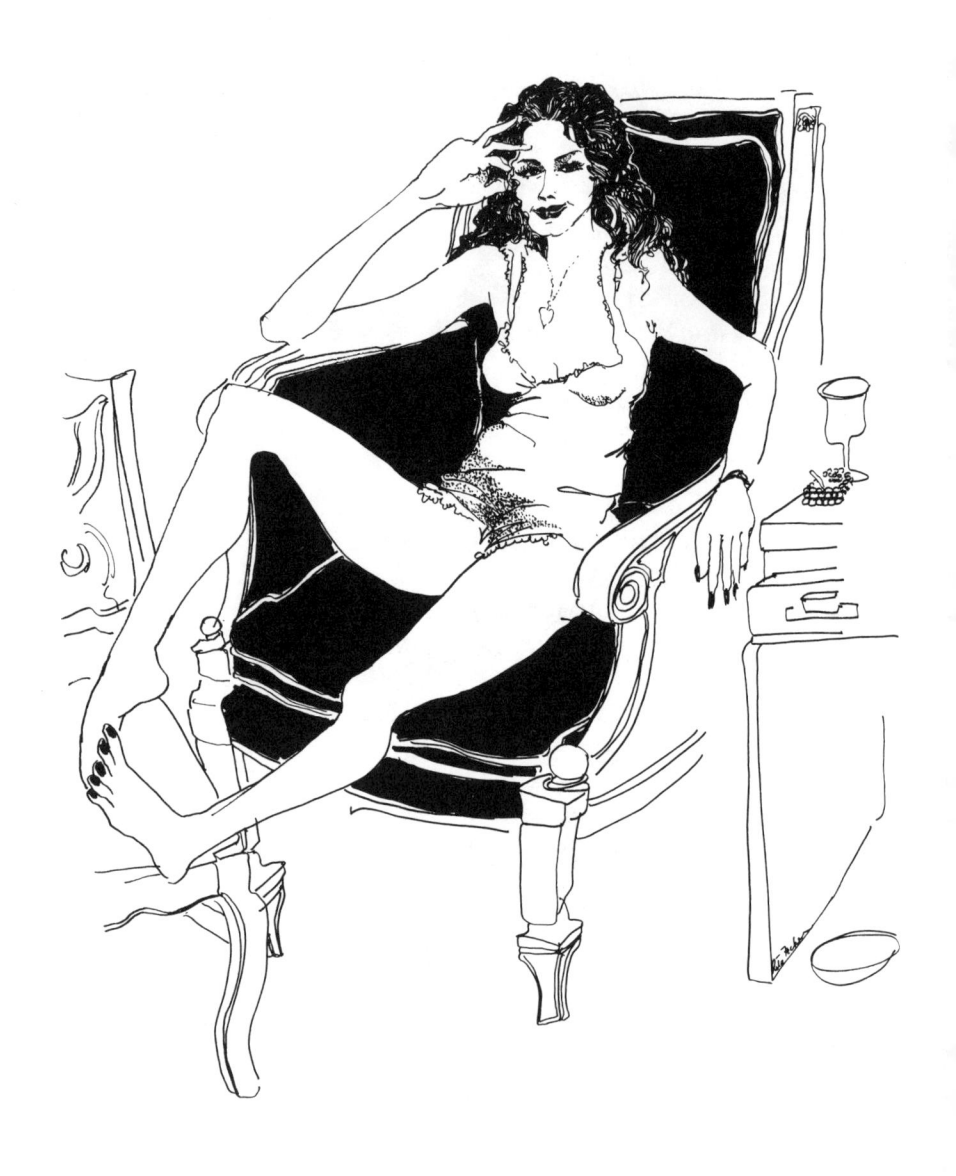

My breasts hurt. They need a massage.

BRAZILIAN
LINES

If you really love me, why don't you have sex with me?

My wife does not understand me.

Our talk is nice; why not have lunch together?

Why should you be offended when I say something nice? I say something nice to make you feel nice. Asking a girl to go to bed with me is a compliment.

Would you like to go to a quiet place?

You're the kind of woman my mother would like me to have.

My breasts hurt. They need a massage.

You're a real woman—not like the kind I have at home.

Will you marry me?

You've never had a lover before me?

How many times have you had love in your life?

JAMAICAN LINES

If you love me, you'll prove your love by having sex with me.

If you don't have sexual intercourse you will get sick.

If you don't have sexual intercourse with me you don't love me.

If you don't have sex with me I will get another girl.

I am yours and nothing can change me.

I cannot get pregnant because I have not lost my virginity yet.

You won't get pregnant the first time you have sex.

You won't get pregnant if we do not discharge together.

You will have headaches or go mad if you do not have sex.

I'll pull out before I come.

If we have sex standing up or in the sea, you can't get pregnant.

I don't box with gloves on.

You are the only one for me.

See white man does it, but doesn't *want us* to.

COLOMBIAN LINES

Sex is an interpretation of love.

If you are not treated well at home, I can give you love.

You are an adult already, you want your independence. I can give you that independence!

I will give you economic security, which you don't have now.

You will not need to work anymore. I will give you all you need; you just give me love.

You like me, I want you, I am in love with you.

I decided that I want to make love with you.

You are really a dream I want for life, really.

May I kiss you?

COSTA RICAN LINES

Prove your love to me.

We will get married.

Now that you have excited me, we must have sex or I will have great pain in my testicles, and I will risk becoming infertile.

I will not do you any harm; I'll come outside of you.

What's the matter, don't you love me?

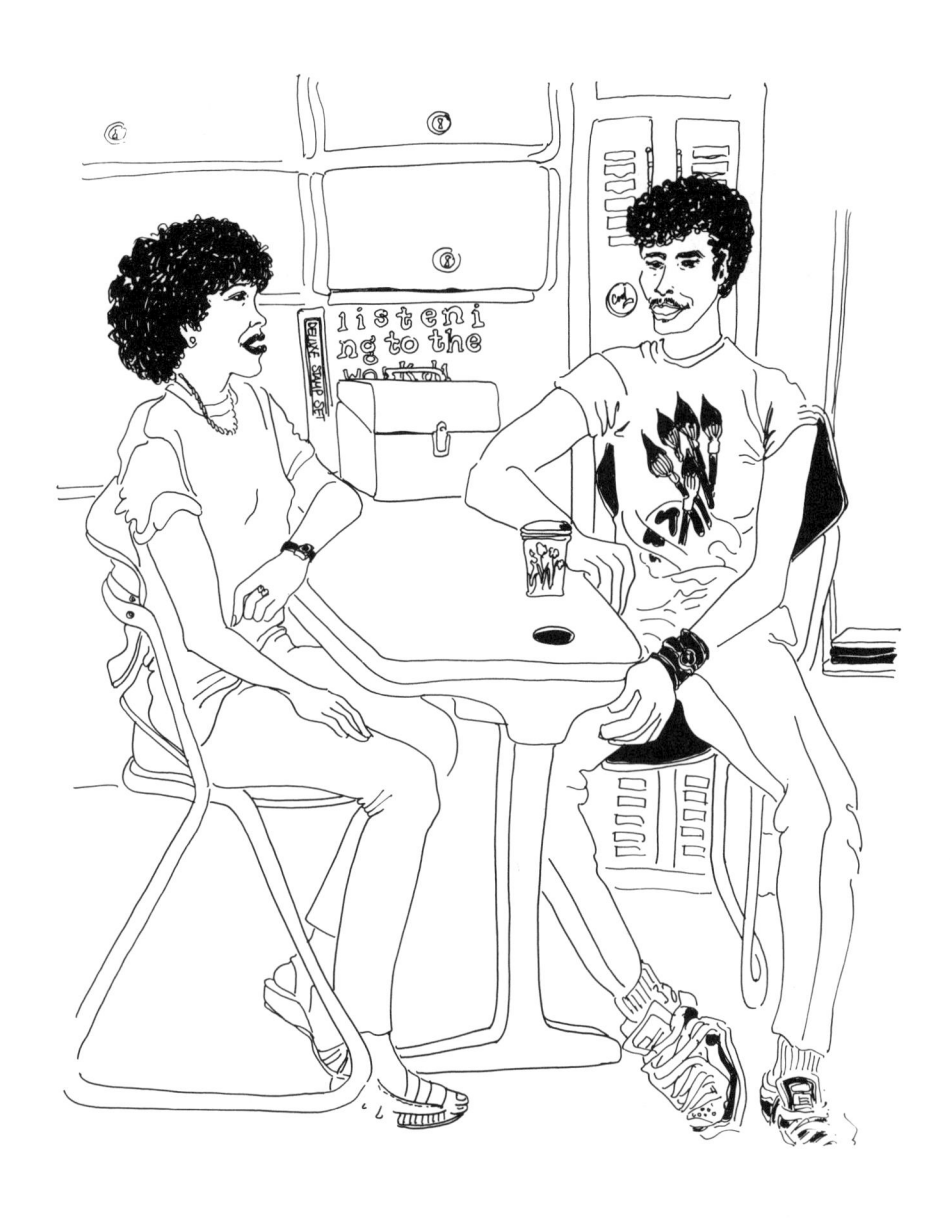

I need to say something very important to you, but it must be in privacy. Do you understand?

URUGUAYAN LINES

Let us go for a drive. I know a beautiful place to see the sunset.

Why you don't come with me to hear the new records I brought from the States?

I need to say something very important to you, but it must be in privacy. Do you understand?

ARGENTINIAN LINES

You know nothing is going to happen, we are just going to caress each other and prove the love we have for each other.

You always leave my balls aching; you can't leave me like that.

Everybody does it, except us.

Think for yourself; don't go by what others tell you.

We aren't kids.

We love each other, so nothing else matters.

I'll have to look somewhere else, with another woman, for what you don't give me. I am a man, and I need to satisfy my sexual instinct.

SALVADOREAN LINES

If you really love me, show it.

Give me the proof of your love.

You'll be mine.

I love you so much that I can hardly resist.

I promise you that we'll be very happy.

I'll do it slowly and gently.

I would like to marry you, but I need you now in this moment.

I would like to be alone with you.

Don't worry, it won't hurt you.

SURINAMESE LINES

If you really love me, you'll have sex with me.

You don't love me if you don't do it with me.

You never get pregnant the first time.

We won't do it for real.

We will be very careful.

You're still a mother's baby.

If you refuse me, it means you're inexperienced.

I did it with others and nothing went wrong.

I promise you it won't hurt.

We won't go all the way.

GRENADIAN LINES

Prove that you love me.

If you don't do it, you will go mad.

Since we love each other, people expect us to have sex.

If you don't do it, you will not be able to talk about the experience with your friends.

If you don't do it, you'll be missing out on life.

The greatest way of expressing love is through sex.

By giving sex you earn yourself more love.

You won't get pregnant.

Nothing is going to happen to you.

I can control myself.

I know when to pull out.

You can't get pregnant now.

I'll die if I don't get it.

TRINIDAD AND TOBAGO LINES

If you love me, prove it.

This will bind us together.

If we have sex, we will know if we are suited for each other.

Sooner or later you'll have to, so you might as well give in now.

You can't keep your cherry forever.

I am taking the pill so you cannot get pregnant.

You have been leading me on, and if we don't have sex my seeds will get blocked up.

If you don't do it, the blood will go to your head.

We are going to be married, so we may as well start now.

It's not modern to be a virgin anymore.

If you don't have sex now, your hymen will turn into cement.

If you don't have sex, the semen will get hard in your back.

Stop behaving like a child. Are you never going to grow up?

You will get sick if you don't have sex at a certain age.

I will buy you a ring tomorrow.

I like your afro hair-do.

You are the only girl who has affected me this way.

You have led me on, and now I'm in terrible pain.

Meet me on Saturday. I want to be with you.

Everybody is doing it, chick.

To love is nothing
To be loved is smaller
To love and be loved
    is everything

ARUBIAN LINES

If you really love me, you'll have sex with me.

First-time opens thirst-time, causes burst-time and fixes birth-time.

AUSTRALIAN LINES

Are you willing to see if we are "compatible"?

What are you keeping it for? It's meant to be used.

Let's behave like liberated adults.

These moral/religious objections really cramp your style.

You must use it once it's up or it's unhealthy.

You've got me to this stage. You can't stop now.

Virginity is another word for frigidity.

Liberated women sleep around and are more fun to be with.

What do you think God put you here for?

If you don't, you must be frigid or a lesbian.

You're a great bush walker!

How about a naughty?

Do you want to die wondering?

Come on, it's fun.

You really want to—the problem is the inhibitions you've inherited from your parents.

What's the matter with you—got a sex problem?

How can we have a totally fulfilling relationship without sex?

I'm as randy as hell.

We must be sexually compatible in order to get along as people.

I've always wanted to lay a spunky bird like you, darling.

TOGOLESE LINES

Prove you really love me.

Your refusal to have sex with me means you love another.

Are we brother and sister to stay without sex?

Don't behave like you were not emancipated.

Is there any love without sex?

In the matter of love, only sex can make you mature.

Are you waiting for your parents' permission to have sex?

Never listen to gossipers; you have to experience sex.

Only an abnormal girl can refuse to have sex with her lover.

Sex is vital for your health.

Sex is a physiological need.

Without sex, I don't know whether I really love you.

It's only through sex that I can measure the degree of your love.

Let me have sex with you, unless you don't love me.

PAPUA NEW GUINEAN LINES

If you really love me, you'll have sex with me.

Have sex to show the real love.

If you don't have sex with me I am going to leave you. I promise you I will not leave you if you have sex with me.

Love is feeling, liking, and wanting a girl, and it must be expressed by making love.

You must have sex with me to show me that you really love me.

GHANIAN LINES

This is the only way to show that you love me.

Don't behave like a child.

Just try it once and see.

You are so beautiful, so don't behave like that.

Nobody will see you do it.

I will really marry you if have sex with me.

Don't worry about pregnancy; I will use a condom.

You are the only one I have in the world.

I promise you anything under the sun if . . .

UGANDAN LINES

What is your name?

You have very pretty eyes.
　Thank you.

I say, let's go to my place.
　That's O.K. I'm not interested.

There is a party at my house.
　Then you have enough people there, you don't need me.

I say, let's go try me out.
　The only thing you're going to try is getting out of my face.

I say, are you waiting for someone?
　Not really, but I'm not interested in your company.

Can I buy you a drink?
　Sure, as long as you buy my boyfriend one.

You're the most beautiful girl in this whole place.
　Yes, I know because my husband thinks so too.

Would you like to dance?
　Yes, come to think of it, let me ask that guy over there.

Every time I see you my heart leaps for joy.
　Be careful, I would not want your heart to jump out of your chest.

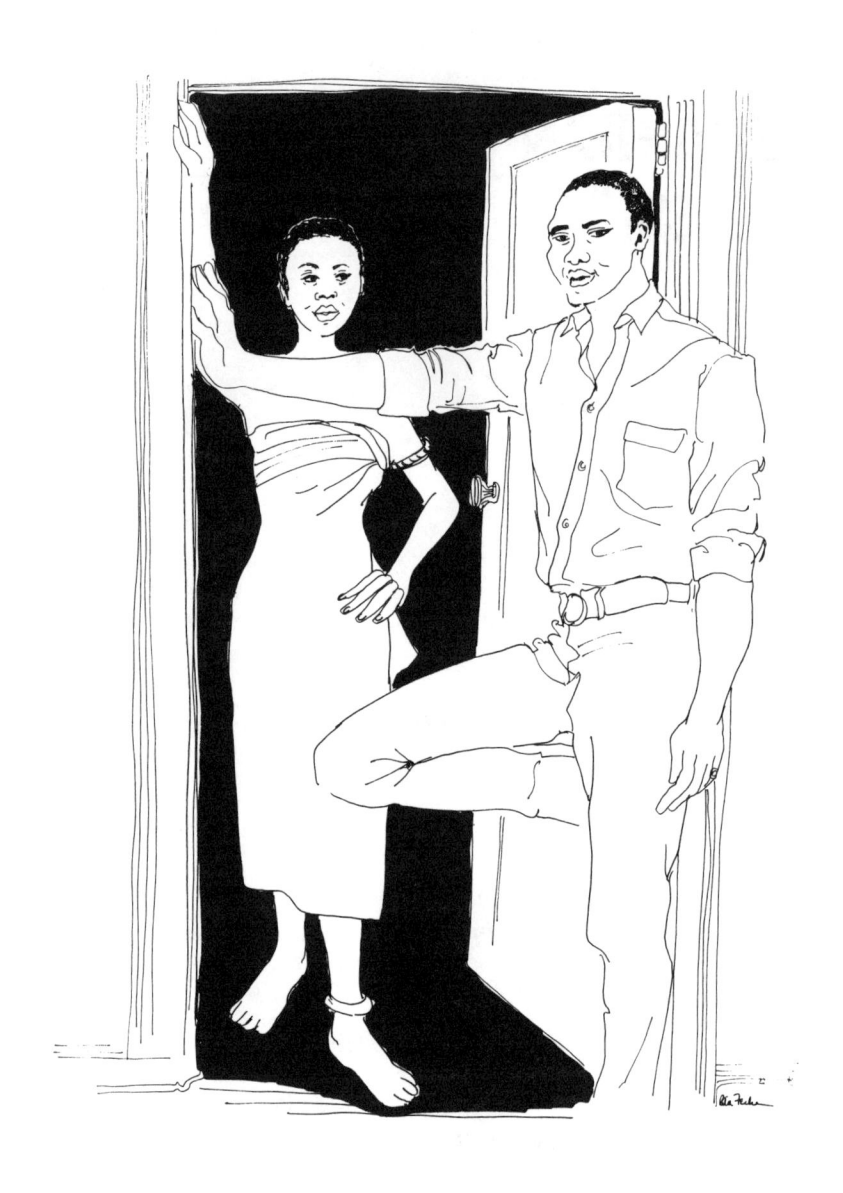

He: I say, let's go try me out.
She: The only thing you're getting is out of my face.

You know how to make a guy sweat between his legs.
Then you must have a bad problem.

Excuse me, would you like to dance?
No.
Then a blow job must be out of the question.

TANZANIAN LINES

Show that you love me; I'm tired of words.

Why don't we go ahead, most modern girls do it. Are you backward or something?

I can't control myself. Help me please!

NIGERIAN LINES

If you are convinced that you love me, why not show me by giving it to me?

Well, I am not going to press you further, but note that if I didn't love you I wouldn't ask you.

It's only a game.

Let me put the penis at the tip of the vagina. I won't go in, I promise.

If you marry me, we'll be the happiest couple in the world.

Don't worry. If you're pregnant, I'll accept full responsibilities.

My father is the richest man in our town.

I always have a stomach upset if I don't get the sexual act.

I will do everything you ask me to do—I will obey you.

I have found that you belong to me.

You are my pet.

We must have met before in the past world.

I am one man, one woman.

You have stolen my heart.

You are my lucky lip.

Why not come home with me? I have two-bedroom apartment.

Miss, can I have the honor of your company on the dance floor?

GAMBIAN LINES

If you love me, let's have sex.

Please give me a chance.

I want to be with you.

My love for you will never die.

You know I love you.

I want to make love with you.

Let's have sex; nobody will know.

I will not make you pregnant.

I will marry you when I make you pregnant.

Let's establish our relationship.

I'll marry you.

Let me taste your sexuality before I decide to marry you.

SIERRA-LEONEAN LINES

If you love me, show me your love.

You cannot get pregnant if we do it standing up.

You are educated; you are liberated. What's your inhibition?

Are you frigid?

Don't worry, baby. I've got a good doctor who has a tablet for you to take. Nothing will happen; I'll take care of you.

Get pregnant, and I shall marry you.

Nothing will happen; I'll take care.

I'll buy all that you have ever wanted.

Let's jazz it up.

I will withdraw.

LIBERIAN LINES

Prove your love.

I will do everything for you once you get pregnant for me.

I will give you a happy life if your parents get rid of you.

Just give me a chance and I will prove 100 percent.

Don't buy pigs in the bag.

Severe headaches mean you are sexually ready.

SUDANESE LINES

I love you, and it is only once and this time.

Oh, my moon, let us have a trip.

Your lips are like a date picked of honey.

ZAMBIAN LINES

If you love me, let me make love to you.

Look, baby, I am head-over-heels in love with you. I need you in order to survive. So come on, let's have it.

You are my food and my very being.

Don't worry, I will withdraw in time so that you won't get pregnant.

Relax please. I will marry you if you get pregnant after this.

Come on! You will enjoy it. There's nothing wrong in making love.

I will be very careful, so please relax, and let me show you what to do.

I won't make you pregnant, as I have never made any other girl pregnant by making love to her.

If you allow me to make love to you, I promise to give you all the financial support you need in the world.

I will marry you if only you can get pregnant for me and prove to be fertile.

If you don't let me make love to you, that will prove that you are not a real woman.

If you don't let me make love to you, then I will leave you for good and go for another girl more sexually active than you are.

You are the most beautiful girl I have ever met. I have met others before, but you are exceptional!

My mother will love you because you have features like hers.

I love you from the bottom of my heart. Please hold me tight and prove it for yourself.

If you become pregnant, I will marry you. Let's produce more soldiers for our motherland. We are underpopulated. How about that, baby?

LESOTHAN LINES

You are all mine and the only one.

I won't take long, just five minutes on the thighs only.

Oh, if I don't do it now, I'll die. I'll be a good boy and not spill inside.

Don't be dumb, most modern girls do it; nobody will know that we have done it.

MAURITIAN LINES

If you really love me, you'll have sex with me.

Life is too short, why not make the most of it?

Most probably there is another guy.

So what? No one else will know.

You are my everything.

I will commit suicide if I cannot make love to you.

You are mine and I am yours.

Come, sweet, the world is ours.

Darling, you are my light. Without you it's darkness.

Sweetheart, you are my heart. Without you I am a dead man.

MALAYSIAN LINES

Marriage is just a piece of paper to make public a very private affair.

I am different from other men. The more sex I have with a woman, the more I love her.

Don't think that marriage is everything. In fact, it is the beginning of trouble and the end of love.

You are luckier being unmarried and getting the best of everything. What is marriage after all, just a routine thing day in and day out?

You are a great girl.

You are such a beautiful girl.

May I touch your hand?

What a sexy girl you are, and what a sexy body too.

You are smart.

You look cute.

You know, you look better without your spectacles.

I never go around with other girls. I love only you.

You are sweet, and I like you very much, and I do not have any other girl friends.

You are the most wonderful of all. You are the most pretty girl I have ever seen.

I am not like other boys; I am different from others.

Why make such a fuss? After all, I am going to marry you soon.

INDONESIAN LINES

If you really love me, you will certainly do it for me.

It is a way of proving your love for me.

Don't be afraid. Sex is something every girl will certainly experience.

We will get married some day, so there are no differences whether we do it now or later.

Don't worry, I will marry you when you get pregnant.

I will suffer if you don't want to do it.

Have a try. I promise not to do anything you don't want.

All your friends have done it.

I don't desire anyone else but you.

INDIAN LINES

It is right and proper for people who truly love each other to give themselves fully to each other.

You're the prettiest girl I've seen, and I'll be proud of you, more so if I can have you.

You know something? You are the only one I love, and am going to love you forever.

You are charming, gentle, and lovely.

You are sexy.

You are pretty.

If you don't make tomorrow's date, then don't blame me if you lose me.

You'd better come tomorrow if you don't want to lose me, as I am nearly losing interest in you.

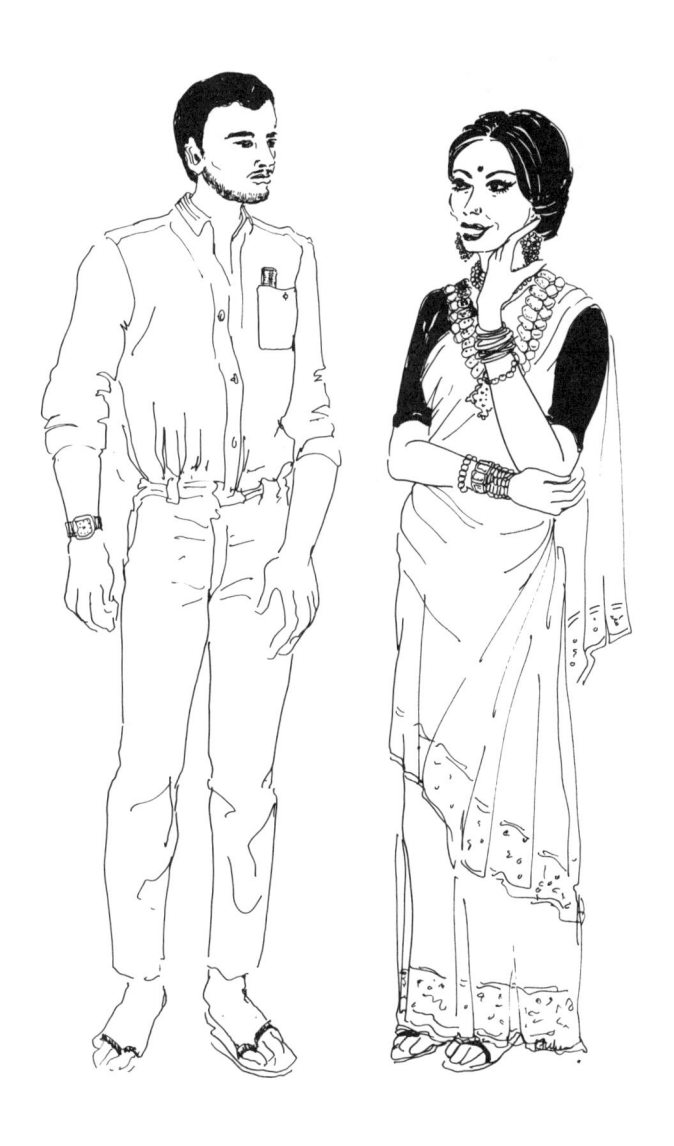

It is right and proper for people who truly love each other to give themselves fully to each other.

LEBANESE LINES

Will you have sex with me?

I am sure this is my lucky day because I met the most beautiful woman in my life.
> *And how many lucky days have you had so far?*

Whenever I see your pretty face, it is like seeing the moon.
> *Oh, but I thought the moon had mountains and valleys.*

Do you know that you brighten my life like a moon brightens a dark day?
> *What do you do when the forecast is cloudy? Look for another planet?*

Oh, darling, I can't imagine my life without you.
> *I can.*

When I am with you, I feel like I own the whole world.
> *Can you give up the part that includes me in it?*

Do you think something can build between us in the future?
> *Yes, the Great Wall of China.*

ARABIC LINES

You would if you loved me.

You make my eyes move.

Your face is beautiful like the moon.

Your cheeks are as beautiful as roses are red.

My love is bigger than the sea is great.

JAPANESE LINES

Can I buy you a drink?

Do you come here often?

Let's have some coffee in the morning.

Shall we change the place?

Let me trip your Toru?

How about driving your bullet train into me?

Let me scale your Mt. Fuji.

Let me pluck your cherry blossoms.

Let me mediate in your Zen.

Do you have the yen?

Would you like to take a drive to the sea with me?
Go yourself, and while you're at it, splash some cold water on your head!

Why don't we go to a darker place for the good thing?
Go there alone and do it yourself.

Let's go to a nice quite place and talk about our future all night.
Sure, if you don't mind my boyfriend coming with us.

You look great in red.
> *Shut-up! Before I show you how good you look in red!*

Would you like to see my new stereo?
> *Why don't you just clean the stupid wax out of your ears?*

I've been thinking of you for a long time.
> *I've been thinking of you too—your bad breath.*

Would you like to go out for tea with me?
> *Are you kidding? Go home and wash your face and maybe then I'll think about it.*

Can I buy you a drink?
> *My mom told me never to accept candy from a stranger.*

Do you mind if I sit next to you?
> *What are you talking about? You? Have you ever seen your face? Here, I'll let you use my mirror!*

Can I take you home?
> *I didn't know you could drive. [A driver's license is very difficult to get in Japan; it can cost up to $700.00.]*

Your smile makes me happy. I want to take you and your smile home with me tonight.
> *Here then, take my picture home!*

SINGAPORESE LINES

The only way you can show your love for me is to give in to me.

My love for you will grow stronger after we have had sex.

If you love me, how can you allow me to suffer as I am now doing—seeing and admiring you, wanting you, and not getting you?

We'll have fun. You'll enjoy it, and no one need know about it.

Everyone's doing it these days, and we'd be foolish not to do it.

Oh it's all right, what matters is only us.

If anything should happen I promise you I will stand by you.

Since we love each other there is no harm in it.

So what have you got to lose? The abortion facilities are always easily available.

If you really love me, you will want to have it with me.

I love you so much and desire you so much that I can't wait to have it with you.

Darling, how about it?

CHINESE LINES

How about it? After all, everyone is doing it.

Would you like to go to _____ for a day? At night, you can sleep on my bed, and I'll sleep on the floor. You should trust me, you know.

Your place or mine?

You will be all right as you are in your safe period.

My love is not fully satisfied unless you give yourself to me.

Sleep in my bed, my girl.

You have a smiling face and a very gentle character.

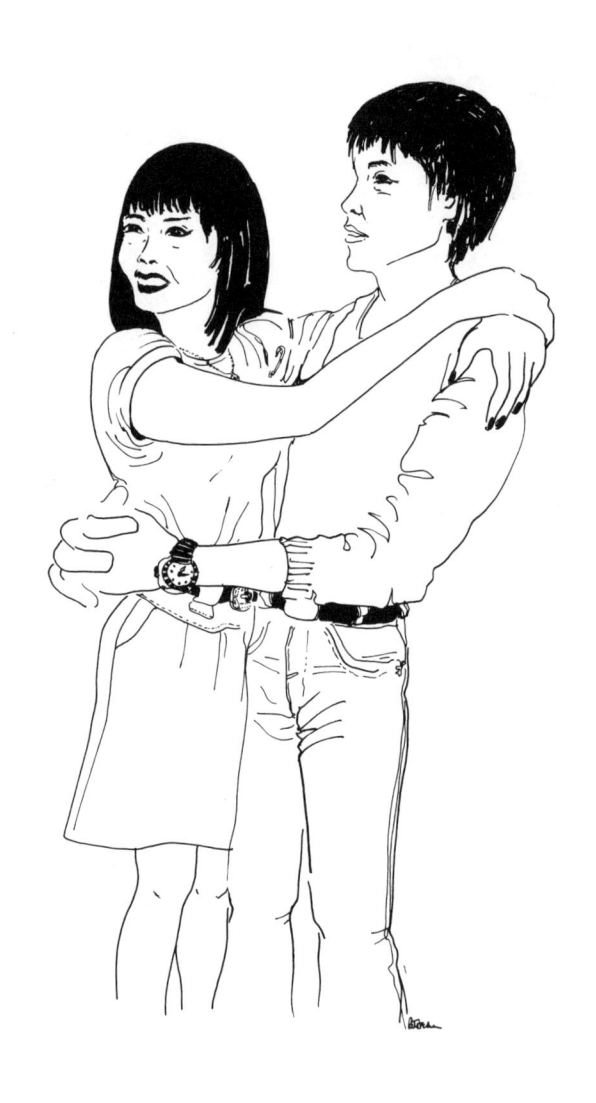

If you really love me, you'll have sex with me.

HONG KONG LINES

If you really love me, you'll have sex with me.

If you love me, you should satisfy my need.

Don't you believe that I will marry you?

Don't be so conservative. This is the twentieth century. It is fashionable to have premarital sex.

Aren't you curious about sex?

We are going to get married anyway. Why can't we have sex now?

What are you afraid of?

You can't understand how desperate I am to have sex.

You'll never know whether we could get along sexually if you don't try it.

It's better for us to find out whether we could get along sexually before our marriage.

You can only start to understand a person after you start to have sex with him. Don't you think so?

You are so sexy and have a nice figure, the best one that I've ever seen among my girl friends.

Let me put my ferry in your Star.

Why wait until 1997 [when Hong Kong reverts to Mainland China]?

Let's get our yin and yang together and bang.

Have you ever seen a one-eyed stalk?

MISCELLANEOUS LINES

THAI LINES

I will marry you and take you for a wife if anything happens.

EGYPTIAN LINES

Don't worry.

SUDANESE LINES

Your lips are like a date picked out of honey.

LIBERIAN LINES

Don't buy pigs in the bag.

I will do anything for you once you get pregnant for me.

EAST AFRICAN LINES

Oh, you look juicy.
    You'll never get to find out how juicy I am.

You are too ripe.
> *That's strange; I'm not in season yet.*

ITALIAN LINES

Ciao, baby. Do you have any Italian in you?
> No.

Would you like some?

I saw you from across the room. You look great tonight.
> *Thanks, but you look better at a distance.*

KOREAN LINES

You really turn me on. Why don't you stay the night with me?
> *Are you crazy, asking me such a thing?*

ISRAELI LINES

Can I give you a private tour?

You know you want it as much as I do.

DANISH LINES

Your place or mine?

ANTIGUAN LINES

I am not marrying a woman unless I am sure that she can have children.

HOW DO YOU SPELL RELIEF?

M-A-S-T-U-R-B-A-T-I-O-N

If it's not right for you to have sexual intercourse, or you are by yourself and you are horny as hell, masturbate yourself or have you and your partner masturbate each other.

Masturbation is a normal and healthy expression of sexuality at any age. Mind you, you can also live a healthy normal life without ever having masturbated. If you don't feel good about masturbation, it is probably because you've been punished or made to feel guilty for doing it.

Masturbation is an almost universal phenomenon. On a voluntary basis, you can't do it too much. However, once is too much if you don't like it. If you don't like it, don't do it.

Like everything else, masturbation can become compulsive (involuntary). There are people who eat too much, not because they are hungry, but because they have high levels of anxiety, and there are people who drink too much alcohol, not because they are thirsty, but again because of tension and nervousness. The same can be true of masturbation.

Now get this: If you absolutely must have a compulsion, please choose masturbation. No one has ever died of over-masturbating, but thousands of people die every year as a result of compulsive eating and drinking. Masturbation is clearly the compulsion of choice. It's cost effective.

THE PUNCH LINE

"I don't wanna" is reason enough not to. People who are secure about their "no"s know when to say "yes." And finally, a response to:

"You would if you loved me."

Reply,

"The truth now: Would you want to even if I didn't love you? I think you would, so what's the point?"

or

"Hey, no more games."

If he says:

"Let's have a good time. And in the process we can figure out if we are meant for each other."

Reply,

"Haven't you discovered that the best way to test a relationship is to see if it works without sex . . . for a long period of time?"

Do you want more information? For a free annotated list of the best sex education books, write to the distributor: Ed-U Press, 7174 Mott Rd., Fayetteville, N.Y. 13066.